fit by na

THE ADVENTX™ TWELVE-WEEK OUT

fit by nature

THE ADVENTX™ TWELVE-WEEK OUTDOOR FITNESS PROGRAM

JOHN COLVER WITH M. NICOLE NAZZARO | PHOTOGRAPHY BY SEAN AIRHART

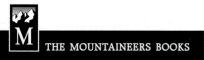

THE MOUNTAINEERS BOOKS

For my mother, Margaret.—J.C.
For my parents, and in memory of Martin Duffy.—M.N.N.

THE MOUNTAINEERS BOOKS
is the nonprofit publishing arm of The Mountaineers Club, an organization founded in 1906 and dedicated to the exploration, preservation, and enjoyment of outdoor and wilderness areas.

1001 SW Klickitat Way, Suite 201, Seattle, WA 98134

Distributed in the United Kingdom by Cordee, www.cordee.co.uk

Manufactured in China

Project editor: Joan Gregory
Copy editor: Kim Runciman
Design: Heidi Smets Graphic Design, heidismets.com
Photographer: Sean Airhart
Cover photography: Sean Airhart
Illustrations: Dennis Arneson
Photographs on pages 44 and 141 by Gudmundur Brynjarsson.

Library of Congress Cataloging-in-Publication Data
Colver, John.
    Fit by nature : the adventx twelve-week outdoor fitness program / by
    John Colver, with M. Nicole Nazzaro.
        p. cm.
    Includes bibliographical references and index.
    ISBN 978-1-59485-353-1
1. Physical fitness. 2. Outdoor recreation. I. Nazzaro, M. Nicole.
II. Title.
    GV481.C649 2011
    613.7—dc22

                                    2010043959

ISBN (paperback): 978-1-59485-353-1
ISBN (e-book): 978-1-59485-354-8

contents

Section 4: Keep Going

Appendixes

acknowledgments

There are many people without whose help and inspiration this book would not have been possible.

John would like to thank, first and foremost, his mother, Margaret, and father, Geoff, for building a foundation for a rich and fulfilling life full of adventures, gifts, and learning, always with the knowledge that both success and setbacks would be met with love, support, and encouragement. To his brother, Keith, a husband, father, and former Parachute Regiment Officer, John wishes to say: "As a paramedic, you've shown me how to care for people, and as a friend and brother you've simply cared for me. I could not have written this book without your support." John's late grandmother, May Colver, godmother Dorothy, and Brian, Nick, and Chris Crouch have also been wonderful sources of support.

Jeff Dossett's contributions to adventX cannot be overstated; he helped finance adventX in its early days and has been a role model of what a leader can and ought to be. The growth of adventX has been in no small part due to Jeff's coaching, encouragement, and commitment.

Medical advisors Wolfgang Brolley and Sally Hara provided expertise in the areas of physical therapy and nutrition. John would also like to acknowledge Stephanie Gundel's extraordinary coaching and leadership; other coaches include Shannon Svege, Ruthie Naranjo, Katie Tavog, Ilga Solveiga, Tiffany Waldburger, Sherry Jaqua, Ryan Scheaffer, and Elia Blumberg-Mrak.

People who have helped significantly to build adventX and to support John's work include Donn Owlsey; Paul Rosser; Kate Austin; Rick Blumberg; Chris Mrak; Phil Ershler; Eric Simonson; George Dunn; Dr. Robert "Brownie" Schoene; Dr. Scott Marshall; Scott Korner; Brian Tschider; Nick Vikstrom; Dan Nelson; Jay Gotteshall; Debbie Reber; Catherine Lavelle; Charlie Davis;

Heather and Martin de Vrieze; Tony Hoskins; Lana Makhanik; David, Mike, and Julie Mayo; Mitzi Alder; Christy Wallace; Jim Thornton; Ward and Boni Buringard; Lana Makhanik; Randy Huntington; Mike Lawson; and Kellie Morrill.

Sean Airhart and Gudmunder Brynjarsson are responsible for the beautiful photographs in the book. Special thanks to models Teri Foley, Debbie Reber, John Quirk, Jen Longtin, Casey Fairchild, and Wendy Werblin.

Nicole wishes to acknowledge the extraordinary editors who have helped to shape her writing career, particularly Amby Burfoot of *Runner's World*; Craig Neff of *Sports Illustrated*; and Cynthia Gorney and Tom Engelhardt. Andor Boeck and his family have been a constant source of love and encouragement, as has the entire Nazzaro family (mom Catherine, brother Bill, sister-in-law Maureen, sister Susie, and brother-in-law Cory) and dear friend Caraway Seed. Martin Duffy and the Duffy-Stieff family have provided more support than words can describe. Toward the end of this book project, Nicole was blessed with a writing position at Intrepid Learning Solutions in Seattle that provided much-appreciated camaraderie in what can often be a lonely profession. Many thanks to Sam Herring, Judy Albers, Mike Tessem, Tyler Whitworth, Sylvia Wallace, and everyone on the Intrepid team for their support. And without running partner and adventX friend Jo Bader, Nicole would never have found Intrepid—or been pushed to succeed on so many long runs.

Finally, both of us would like to acknowledge the many contributions of Kate Rogers, Editor in Chief at the Mountaineers Books, who first helped envision this book; our agent, Joy Tutela, of the David Black Literary Agency; our project editor, Joan Gregory; copy editor Kim Runciman; and the entire staff of the Mountaineers Books. Kate in particular coached us through every aspect of this book's development, from the first outline to the final proofs. Every project needs a champion, and Kate has championed this book.

John Colver and M. Nicole Nazzaro
Seattle, Washington

foreword

At 9:10 AM Nepal time on May 22, 2004, I stepped onto the summit of Mount Everest, becoming the third Canadian in history to reach the top of each of the highest peaks on every continent, the so-called Seven Summits. At that moment, I felt a sense of personal accomplishment on a level I had never previously experienced.

I wanted to share the moment with John Colver, my coach, business partner, and dear friend, so I dug into my backpack, pulled out my adventX summit banner, and proudly posed for photographs. I spent the next ninety minutes on the summit reflecting on the scope and significance of the personal journey that had culminated in me standing at the top of the world.

It was a transformation of mind, body, and purpose, and I cannot overstate the role that John Colver and adventX, the outdoor fitness company he founded in Seattle, played in inspiring, enabling, and empowering that transformation.

Four years before the Everest summit, I had been at least twenty-five pounds overweight. It had been over twenty years since I had pursued any athletic or fitness goal of any significance, and I instinctively knew that I needed a change in my lifestyle. At forty years old, I was feeling the effects of years working in a fast-paced and stressful work environment.

I first met John Colver when I joined a guided climbing expedition on Aconcagua, the highest mountain in South America at 22,983 feet. John was one of two professional mountain guides leading our expedition team, and we quickly became friends, sharing a passion for mountain climbing, physical and mental challenges, storytelling, and a surprisingly similar, quirky sense of humor.

During our three-week expedition, we encountered a particularly fierce and unexpected snowstorm at about 19,500 feet. For several days, our expedition team was pinned down in our tents as the snow fell heavily. During the storm, John and I passed the time resting, recovering, reading books, and sharing stories in our two-person tent, and that was when I first articulated my "big, bold goal" to complete the Seven Summits. I had taken a much-needed break from my full-time career in the software and technology business to focus on improving work/life balance, in large part by pursuing a completely different and intensely challenging personal goal. I remember distinctly how supportive and enthusiastic John was as I shared my Seven Summits dream.

John, too, was at a crossroads. He had enjoyed a rich and varied set of life experiences, ranging from military service, working as a certified wilderness EMT, competing nationally as an elite cyclist, and acting as a senior mountain guide, to assuming leadership roles in sales and marketing at a principal North American bike manufacturer. Yet he too seemed to yearn for a new and different challenge—to pursue his own "big, bold goal": to establish an outdoor fitness company that reflected his passion for nature and his belief that the outdoors gives us all we need to attain complete fitness.

During that storm, John and I committed ourselves to getting serious about making specific plans and progress against our goals. The idea for adventX had percolated in John's mind for some time, but I'd like to believe that our discussion was a turning point for him. John found strength of purpose and motivation in my confidence in his concept. I found someone who inherently believed that I could achieve my dream.

At the "Our Team" section of the adventX website (www.adventx.com), you'll find that I'm listed as a "co-founder" of adventX. To say I'm a co-founder of adventX is to gain insight into the core of John's character and integrity; it is a reflection of the magnanimous person he is. A freak snowstorm put us in a tent together high on a mountain in South America. I was simply present, yet I believe that we were uniquely receptive to each other's dreams and enthusiasm in that moment. Perhaps as important was our willingness to be honest enough with each other to share the fears and obstacles that had held us back from realizing the full potential of our dreams to that point.

In this book, John will share the information to help you create your own outdoor fitness program. It's a unique blend of concepts, approaches, methods, techniques, and plans—all fueled by defining personally relevant goals and sources of motivation. I used to have goals like "be in the best shape of my life," "lose some weight," "be more active," or "get out more." With John's guidance and support, I quickly realized that those weren't goals, they were dreams. He will help you translate your dreams into explicit (often transformational) goals supported by specific training plans and metrics that enable you to measure your progress. Only then can you convert your dreams into your willed future.

I am a different and better person for my association with John Colver and his extraordinarily successful adventX outdoor endurance fitness experience. Over the past six years, I have witnessed hundreds of adventX team members achieve personal transformations that exceeded even their highest expectations. To me, fitness enables an active and healthy lifestyle. John Colver and his method showed me the path and gave me the knowledge, tools, and techniques to transform my lifestyle. With the support of my adventX family, today I have new dreams, which I am in the process of converting into goals and a new willed future. Take the first step. Join me; join the adventX community.

Jeff Dossett
Woodinville, Washington

—*Jeff Dossett is a former Microsoft and Yahoo! executive, Seven Summits mountaineer, two-time Mount Everest summit climber, and adventX athlete.*

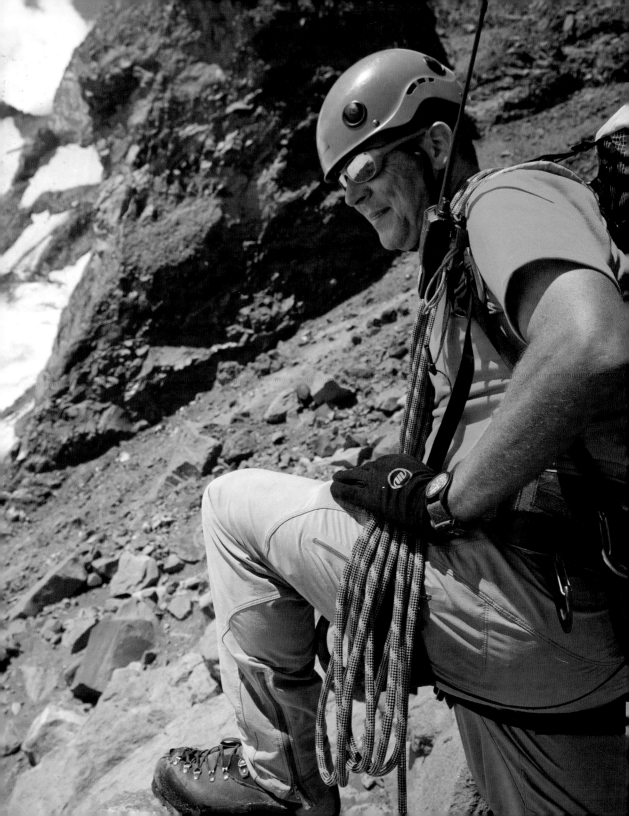

how the outdoors will change your life

Follow your dreams always. You will live once and I want you to know that your adventures are not frivolities. They will be the pivotal junctions of your life.

—May "Gran" Colver, 1917–2009

Nature is a profound place. The outdoors offer an experience of vast richness with endless possibilities for personal growth. This book invites you into a beautiful and limitless playground, a place where you can attain a level of fitness you may never have thought possible, all by walking outside your front door. You can create a fantastic workout routine in the outdoor spaces that surround you. It doesn't matter if you live in a bustling city, rural farmland, or something in between. It only matters that you want to change your life by bringing your workout program into the natural world.

The outdoors have been an integral part of my life. Growing up in Scotland, I was a national cycling champion and served as an officer and paratrooper in the elite Parachute Regiment of the British Army. I trained exclusively in outdoor settings, and got to know firsthand the opportunities that the outdoor world provides us for reaching our fitness goals. We never had a gym available to us, so to speak; instead, the world was our gym. Hiking and climbing in the spectacular Scottish Highlands and the Alps, riding up famous French mountain passes like the Col de Tourmalet and Mount Ventoux, where champions past and future had toiled in pursuit of their dreams, were all a part of a rich experience of outdoor fitness adventures.

In the early stages of writing this book, someone asked me, "Where do you work out?" My answer was simple: "Wherever I want." Most often, it's outdoors. The outdoors have given me a sense of complete freedom in my physical training, because the possibilities for training are just about limitless. And because being outdoors means being surrounded by beautiful settings, it's where I want to be most of the time.

Why do it? Why punch an alarm clock early in the morning and go outside for a workout? Simply put, the outdoor fitness lifestyle will change your life in ways you may never have imagined. Whether you're zipping up your rain jacket, pulling on a hat and gloves on a cold day, or relishing the warmth of a summer's morning, you'll know you're about to see friends and go through your workout routine. You'll feel the cleanness of the air, the softness of the grass, the warmth of the sun, and the sounds of the dawn. Birds chirping, leaves in the breeze, breath, laughter, and company—and maybe even a splash of oars from a boater on a nearby lake. These are the sounds of your everyday workout space—a pretty cool place to be any day of your life. There's nothing better.

My goal in writing this book is for you to use it to further knowledge you already have, or for you to follow this program and use the tools, ideas, and inspiration I have found in the simple act of exercising outdoors. The concepts are based on the award-winning adventX training program I founded in Seattle. The name "adventX" is pronounced "ad-vent-ex" and it stands for "adventure exercise." That is what this book offers you: a way to exercise and have great adventures at the same time, right outside your front door.

The core values of our training program are encompassed by our motto, "Adventure, Fitness, Community."

Adventure: This program gives you the tools to have an extraordinary experience of exploration in the natural world as you get fit. You'll learn how to set your own goals and move toward them with strength, enthusiasm, and a deep confidence in the probability of your own success and excellence. The word "adventure" conveys a sense of goals that may be bigger than you might otherwise be comfortable with—at least at first. But rest assured, as you work through this program, you'll learn how to set truly adventurous goals.

Fitness: This program will help you get fit. In fact, you might say that your fitness is guaranteed with this program—as long as you persevere. Expect success: you're already taking the right course of action by reading this book. How you feel about that, your expectations, visualizations, and positive thoughts as you move toward a new fitness lifestyle are all part of making your fitness journey a successful one.

Community: Even though our society promotes self-reliance, our experience is that having a group of friends or a social network of like-minded people is an important—if not the *most* important—aspect of success in creating a fit, healthy lifestyle. There truly is strength in numbers. The workouts you'll discover in this book can be done alone or with a group of people of all abilities, from beginning athletes to people who are positively addicted to their sports. Get together with friends or a group for a workout, and see if you don't automatically feel inspired. If you prefer to work out alone, that's absolutely fine; a group is not at all required for this workout routine. The key strength of this program is that it is adaptable to your location, circumstances, and lifestyle.

Before we get started, I want to ask one thing of you. See yourself as an athlete from this day forward, no matter what your current level of fitness is. We are all athletes. Of course, there are differences between gold-medal Olympians and the rest of us, but imagine the Boston Marathon race leader charging to the finish line, heart pumping, muscles straining, with a clarity of focus so great that nothing else matters. Is this not exactly the same feeling you will have as you push out your last set of stair climbing, as you feel your heart race as you complete an adventX-style workout? The answer is *yes*. The level of achievement may be different, but the amount of effort expended, and the physical and mental rewards that come with the accomplishment, are just as rich.

As coaches, we watch people make life-affirming decisions every day. In an uncertain world, our physical fitness is one sure gift we can claim. It costs almost nothing, and it pays out freely. In this book, you'll learn that the world outside your door is the only gym you'll ever need, but even more valuable, you'll discover that everything you need to succeed is already within you. Think of our time together as an exploration of your own potential. Be prepared to be amazed at what you can do.

John Colver
Seattle, Washington
john@adventx.com

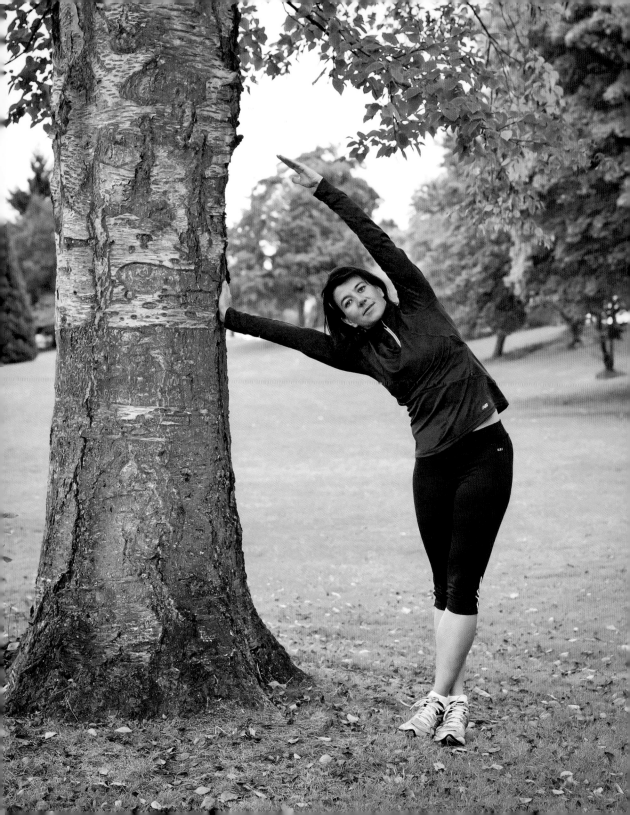

A NOTE FROM CO-AUTHOR M. NICOLE NAZZARO

This program will challenge you in a way that won't just be physique changing, or even fitness changing. It might just be life changing. I come to this book both as a co-author and as a success story. About three years ago, I had the opportunity to try out one of John's outdoor training classes with a friend, after many weeks of hearing her rave about the workouts. Very quickly, I realized this program would both give me a new perspective on what it means to be an athlete in a natural surrounding, and it would, to put it politely, kick my butt.

And it did. As I write these words, I'm far fitter than I used to be, running road races faster than I did ten years ago, when I thought I was as fit as I would ever be. "Athlete" is not the word I would have used to describe myself when I first started working with John. Desk-jockey writer with too many extra pounds around my midsection—that was more like it. I still do tons of writing and sit down quite a lot while doing it, but that's not the part of my life that defines me any longer. The adventX program turned me into an athlete, and that's a priceless feeling.

So join us as we introduce you to the world that John has lived in for all of his life, a world that I entered just a few short years ago and now can't live without. The outdoors will provide you with an amazing gymnasium, full of wonder and adventure, no matter whether your playground is a backyard, Central Park, or the Rocky Mountains. Wherever you are, you can use the concepts outlined here to inject a whole new level of excitement into your fitness lifestyle. If you're starting from scratch, go for it! Getting outside will change your life. If you're a big-time athlete, the program will keep you challenged as you work toward your next goal. And if you're somewhere in between, you can use these workouts both to challenge yourself and to get your friends and family out there with you, everyone exercising side by side, each person at their own level, pushing themselves as hard as they want.

Whatever your goals, when you venture into the outdoors, we'd love to hear from you about your discoveries. Look us up at www.adventx.com. If you're ever in Seattle, come join us for a class in one of the city's gorgeous parks. And don't ever give up on your fitness goals, no matter what. I'm just one of many, many people whose lives have changed immeasurably for the better as a result of John's program. I look forward to seeing you out there.

M. Nicole Nazzaro
Seattle, Washington
mnicolenazzaro@gmail.com

how to use this book

The first third of this book provides basic information on the program you're about to embark on, including specific chapters on gear, nutrition, injury prevention, and a set of exercises called the Daily Dozen, which I use with all of our athletes for general conditioning. You'll also see a stretching routine we normally use at the end of our workouts—hence its name, the Home Stretch.

To get started, read the opening sections all the way through, or just skim the chapters that have the most relevance for you. Start by familiarizing yourself with the "Daily Dozen" and the "Home Stretch," as these are very important parts of the overall program. Spend a bit of time on the chapter "Training Outdoors, Training by Season" as well, in order to get an idea of the types of workouts you'll be doing and the amount of time you'll need for each of the workouts. Finally, make sure that you have good gear, especially if you're venturing outside during a particularly cold or hot time of year. Your outdoor experiences will be most enjoyable as long as you have the right gear and you've protected yourself from the elements.

While you're looking at the opening chapters, take time to read through "Challenge by Choice: Setting Goals" in the "Preparation" chapter. This will introduce you to our philosophy of goal setting and introduce you to tools we use to help adventX team members visualize and reach their own goals. From there, complete the "adventX On-Target Questionnaire" in Appendix C. You'll refer back to it after you've completed your first twelve weeks of the program, and I think you'll be amazed both at the progress you make in that short period and the ways in which your goals become bigger and more tangible as you experience progress in your fitness.

At that point, you'll be ready to delve into the twelve weeks of workouts. Take time to review each week's workouts the week before you embark upon them, so that you can plan when you will work out and where. This will be especially important in the first few weeks. As your program progresses, you'll get used to each workout, allowing you to spend less time reviewing before heading outdoors.

The exercises used throughout the book are described and illustrated in "The Basic Workouts" chapter or in Appendix A: "Compendium of Exercises." At the beginning of Appendix A is an alphabetical index of all the exercises, telling on what page each is described and illustrated. Initially, you will need to turn to the exercise descriptions and illustrations, to learn how to perform each. After a while, however, you will know the key exercises by heart and they will become part of your daily and life routine.

As you begin, know this: the program is simple and straightforward, but there may be quite a few exercises that are new to you, so please remember to have patience with yourself. Normally, it takes most people several weeks to really adapt to the workouts, especially the longer "Cornerstone Workout." During the first few weeks, it's important to listen to your body and to be patient. Most adventX athletes report that they start seeing big gains in their fitness around week five or six. This is not a "quick fix" program. It is a transitional, life-affirming process that may change the way you feel about your own limits. As you begin, try your best, and do only what feels comfortable to you. Soon you'll feel yourself progressing and becoming much more familiar with what each workout week brings, and that will make it possible to experience even more progress.

The last third of the book gives more instruction about what to do after you've completed the initial twelve weeks of workouts, as well as information on getting the most from your outdoor workout program. You'll find additional resources on the topics covered in this book in the appendixes at the back of the book.

Above all, as you delve into the book, have fun! Being in the outdoors is an experience of great joy and happiness for me and for many others, and I think you'll have much the same experience as you venture outside. Above all: Don't doubt your ability. Doubt your limits. Good luck and train smart.

A NOTE ABOUT SAFETY

Safety is an important concern in all outdoor activities. No book can alert you to every hazard or anticipate the limitations of every reader. The descriptions of techniques and procedures in this book are intended to provide general information. This is not a complete text on exercise techniques. Nothing substitutes for formal instruction, routine practice, and plenty of experience. When you follow any of the procedures described here, you assume responsibility for your own safety. Use this book as a general guide to further information. Under normal conditions, excursions into the outdoors require attention to traffic, road and trail conditions, weather, terrain, the capabilities of your party, and other factors. Keeping informed on current conditions and exercising common sense are the keys to a safe, enjoyable outing.

—The Mountaineers Books

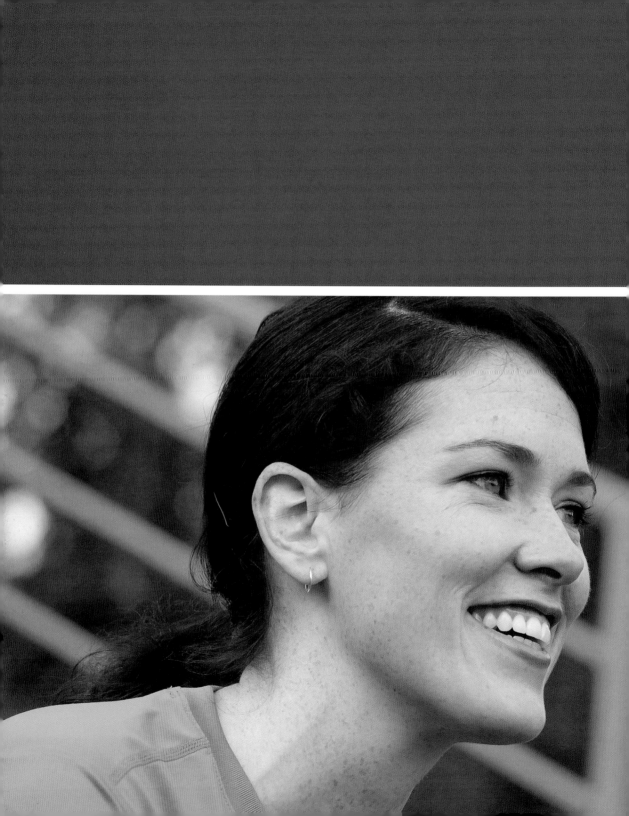

get ready

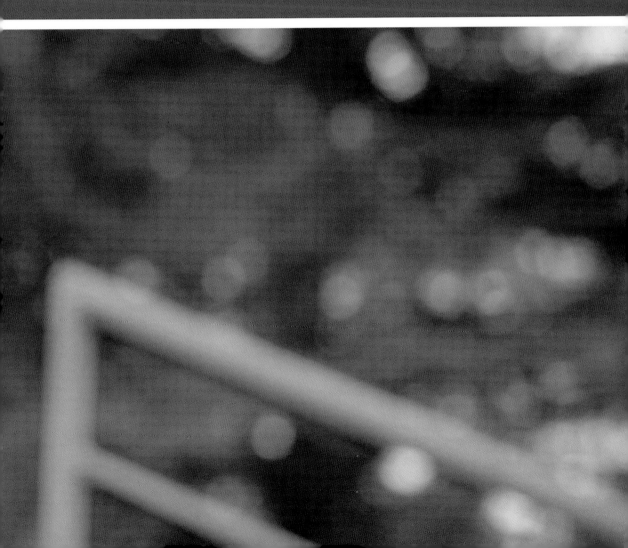

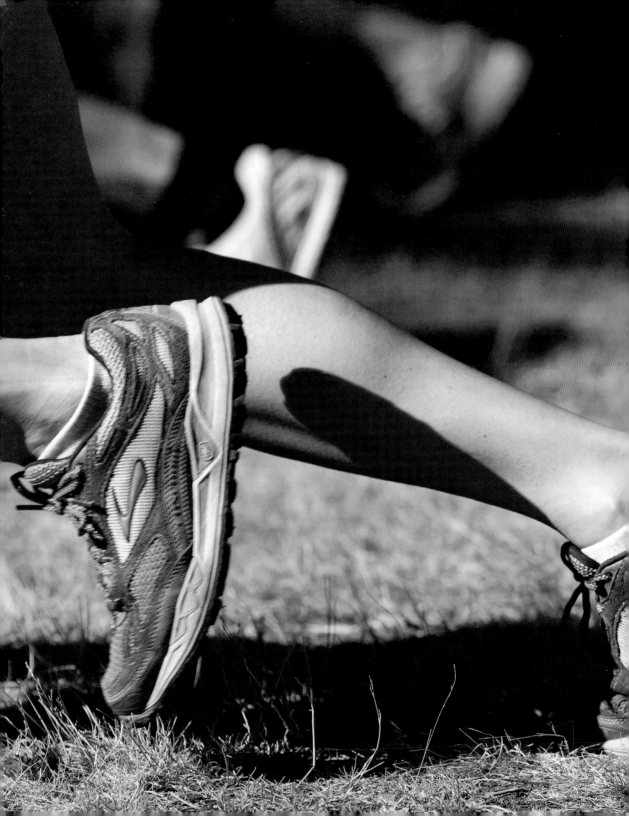

the starting blocks

Fit by Nature is based on solid athletic principles and time-tested philosophies. Week by week, you'll learn a new aspect of training to incorporate into your fitness regimen, and over the full twelve weeks, you'll be amazed at how quickly your body adapts to these new concepts. A daily routine of exercise, restoration, relaxation, good nutrition, and injury prevention will all become part of your new fitness lifestyle.

This program has already been adopted by hundreds of athletes to help vastly improve their base fitness and achieve goals they formerly thought impossible. In one season of training, a thirty-four-year-old woman who had never broken five hours in a marathon clocked 3:47—almost ninety minutes faster than her previous best. She also took twenty minutes off her best half-marathon time. That's just one example of the kinds of improvements in physical performance that our athletes have experienced.

Is it really possible to experience such dramatic gains in the space of a single calendar year? My answer is unequivocal: *Yes. Yes. Yes.* I've seen it happen time and time again as a result of committed, consistent, and moderate training, especially when the athlete has a specific goal in mind.

There are four central tenets, or "starting blocks," to the adventX program, the big picture concepts that make adventX different from any other workout program you've tried. Week by week, you'll add to your fitness knowledge using these key concepts as your anchors. Sidebars will offer more detailed training information.

STARTING BLOCK 1: EXERCISE *OUTDOORS*

The adventX workouts are meant to be done *outdoors*. There are many benefits to training outdoors. One that works beautifully—and that's very similar to the way the best athletes in the world train—is that by training outdoors, you can plan your training by the season. In this book, you'll find a complete twelve-week workout plan, but in reality, as a yearlong athlete, you'll be able to complete a twelve-week cycle, rest and renew for a week, and then move into another seasonal twelve-week cycle with new goals. Four complete cycles of training will give you a full calendar year of workouts and a number of ideas for linking your training to the seasons as you continue to develop your outdoor fitness lifestyle.

Nature is both limitless and complete. You can look up at the sky and see infinite possibilities, and you can survey the terrain and see everything you need for a fitness program. If you're reading this book indoors, the walls and ceilings that surround you can make it hard to imagine the power of the outdoors as an arena for achieving your fitness goals. Don't put artificial ceilings on your goals. In the outdoors, you literally broaden your horizons as you work toward your fitness dreams. Embrace going outdoors as often as you can—and rest assured that this book will help you prepare for the outdoors in every way. By the end of this program, you will feel and act like an outdoor athlete—and you will never look back.

STARTING BLOCK 2: HAVE *FUN*

AdventX is a *fun* workout. You'll work hard, but you'll also have a great time as you move toward your fitness goals. In these pages, you'll find ideas for many new exercises that are meant to be fun as much as they're meant to increase your balance, speed, or strength. The best exercise program is the one you're actually going to do, so be sure to choose the activities that most appeal to you. You may just find that you've forgotten you're exercising and that you are completely engrossed in the activity and in your surroundings. That's a great way to ensure you'll stay interested in your fitness program and keep at it long enough to obtain results.

STARTING BLOCK 3: *CHALLENGE BY CHOICE*

AdventX uses the concept of *Challenge by Choice.* Your workout is under your own control; you'll never be asked to do more than you can do at that moment. You'll train at the level you're comfortable with, never pushing yourself past the point where you become physically exhausted and unable to continue, or past a point where training becomes so all encompassing that you don't have time to live your life. It's all about *moderation* and *consistency,* practiced over a long period of time.

Challenge by Choice puts all the power in your hands to decide how much you want to push yourself on a given day. You always have the choice to do what you think is right: if the book says to do ten repetitions of an exercise, you can do five repetitions—or fifteen. The key is to pay attention to what your body tells you on that day. In time, your body will adapt and crave more movement. The bottom line is this: you can always trust your own body.

Challenge by Choice emphasizes your own involvement and responsibility in the process of becoming an athlete. A big part of completing this program involves learning about your body and how it works best. In short, trust yourself: commit to not pushing yourself past where you want to go on a particular day, in a particular workout. Be your best coach by starting with compassion and a strong belief in yourself.

STARTING BLOCK 4: *VARIETY*

AdventX builds workout weeks around *variety*—of exercises, workout styles, and terrains—to ensure that you're never bored and that your body is always challenged by doing something new. Your most important, and longest, workout of the week is called the **Cornerstone Workout**. You'll also have two to three shorter workouts each week that encompass faster motion to build strength (your **Circuit Training** workouts) and endurance (your **Tempo Workouts**). There will be a daily exercise regimen called the **Daily Dozen**, made up of simple exercises you can do anywhere, as well as a strong self-care component to the program that includes solid nutrition, rest and relaxation, and injury prevention.

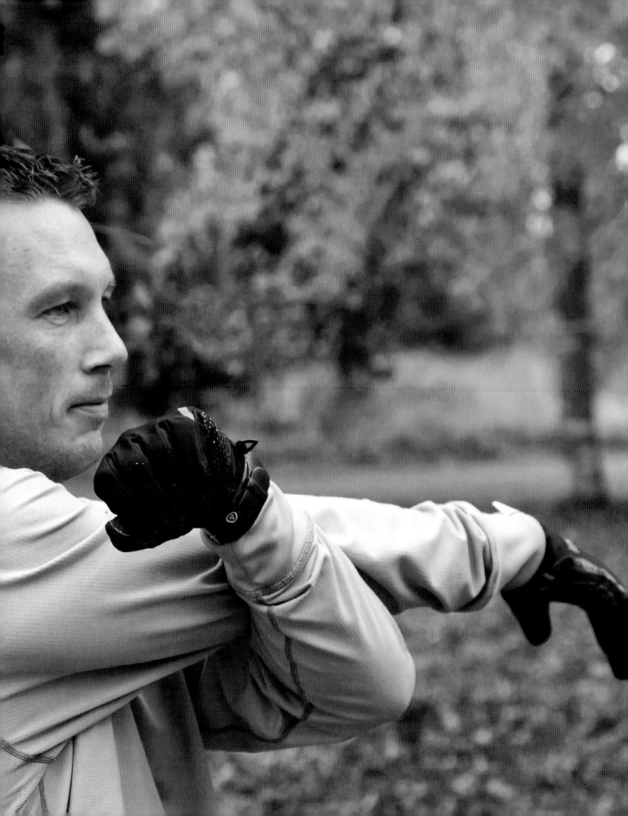

training outdoors, training by season

The outdoors are available to you year-round, at no cost except that of your workout gear. The air is fresh, and the ground is cleaner than in most gyms (after all, how many germs might be on that exercise machine that's been used all week by hundreds of sweaty people?). And it's available to you 24/7. The terrain is varied and unpredictable, and it's physically beautiful, especially if you can find a lakefront, park, or hiking trail.

The twelve-week workout program presented in this book is part of a seasonal fitness plan in which you build up to a peak fitness level every twelve weeks, rest for one week, and then set new goals and embark on a new twelve-week cycle.

For an athlete beginning a workout program in January, the four cycles could look like this:

- **Winter** (January through March): Adapting
- **Spring** (April through June): Building
- **Summer** (July through September): Peaking for top performance
- **Autumn** (October through December): Transitioning

Of course, if you're beginning this program at a different time of year, you can adapt these training cycles to match your own program. When starting an outdoor exercise program for the first time, you may replicate your efforts for more than one season in order to master your skills and awareness, especially if you have not exercised before. That's absolutely fine. The guidelines above are meant to give you a sense of what a seasonally based training program looks like.

THE SEASONS

Each season offers particular benefits for training outdoors. In nature, change is natural—powerful, quick, positive. It's the same with human beings. We may find ourselves stuck in a rut when we've stayed indoors for too long, going through the motions of our workdays. Staying indoors can rob us of energy and imagination. The mere act of going outside and taking in the fresh air can be enough to move us in a more positive direction. And that can lead you to reach for extraordinary achievements. When we say "the sky's the limit," we really mean it.

The season that appears on its face to be the most challenging for outdoor exercise is winter. Let's start there.

WINTER (JANUARY THROUGH MARCH): ADAPTING

WEATHER FACTORS
Dark, cold, wet, possibly snowy.

MOODS
Dark, cold, sleepy, energy level potentially lower.

OUTDOOR TRAINING OPPORTUNITIES
Restorative, invigorating, a breath of fresh air.

Less daylight and more inclement weather do not prevent outdoor training. The overall energy of this time of year, however, is markedly different from the summer. Winter evenings might be spent relaxing, stretching, cooking, studying, planning summer adventures, or making training plans. The overall energy of activities tends to be restorative. (If you're a skier, snowboarder, or snowshoer, you'll be outside in the daylight hours, but nights are still dark and long, so your energy level could be lower than in summer.)

A restorative season allows us to focus on exercises that build strength and flexibility, and help our body adapt to the needs of a new year. Use this time for self-care activities: medical checkups, massage, and other self-care tasks. Given the realities of winter in much of the country, you may plan to exercise indoors when the weather is just too extreme. As a cyclist, I used a

what about weather?

Weather is a definite consideration when deciding whether to go outdoors for a workout or stay inside and adapt your program to that environment. First, you may decide to forego an outdoor workout in excessively cold or icy conditions, in a driving rain, or when it's just too hot outside. You can always adapt this program for the indoors: go to a gym for a cardiovascular workout, or run up and down the stairs in your apartment or office building, or do calisthenics in front of the TV. What I ask is this: don't let the weather stop you if a good rain jacket or other gear will get you going. We hold adventX classes year-round, but Seattle's winters and summers are generally mild, so that's realistic for us. If you're in New York City during a major snowstorm or in Houston in the heat of midsummer, adapt the workout to your own environment. Get outside as much as you possibly can (consult the section "Workout Attire by the Season" in the "Preparation" chapter to make sure you're well protected), but if the weather presents a safety concern or is just too foul, then by all means, work out indoors.

gym for strength training in winter—but I still biked, walked, or ran to that gym whenever possible. All of the activities described in this book can be adapted for use indoors when necessary.

SPRING (APRIL THROUGH JUNE): BUILDING

WEATHER FACTORS
Days get longer, flowers begin to bloom, mixed weather eventually warms up.

MOODS
Awakening, renewing, embracing possibility.

OUTDOOR TRAINING OPPORTUNITIES
A time to get outside and embrace the new season with renewed core strength, flexibility, and stability. Longer endurance workouts will be possible

as the days lengthen, and that focus on endurance will serve you well as you move into a period of getting ready to peak in the summer.

Spring is a great time to really get out of the house, gym, or office. A well-spent winter will have resulted in great core strength, stability, and flexibility, along with a new skill or two. We will have recovered from nagging injuries and become even more aware of how our bodies strengthen and recuperate.

Physiologically, we build endurance in the spring. You can lengthen your weekend workouts, especially the longer endurance workout we prescribe in the twelve-week program. Work on this goal in moderation, gradually adding more time to your longer endurance workout each week to ensure you stay healthy and protect yourself from injury. (A general guideline would be to add no more than 10 percent more time to your longer endurance workout each week.) If you're training for endurance events such as a 10-kilometer race, spring is a time to try a shorter race—perhaps a 5K—to test your fitness and get used to the level of preparedness needed for longer efforts later in the year.

SUMMER (JULY THROUGH SEPTEMBER): PEAKING

WEATHER FACTORS
Sunny, warm to hot (depending on your location).

MOODS
Endless possibility. Virtually no chance of getting stuck indoors by bad weather, except for the occasional summer thunderstorm. Lots of sunshine and long days allow you to feel your best.

OUTDOOR TRAINING OPPORTUNITIES
Full days, all the better to help us achieve the peak of our physical efforts.

Summer is the season when many people plan outdoor adventures. These are often "peak" events—running a race, doing a multiday hike or climb, or taking a vacation related to favorite outdoor activities. Accordingly, we plan the adventX program around the idea of hitting a fitness peak in the summer months. For most of us, it's simply the easiest time of year in which to exercise.

Your summer fitness program will emphasize the skills you're looking to develop for your chosen summer activities. This may include altering your endurance workouts. A hiker who has previously been running and swimming for her longer endurance workout, for example, will likely substitute hikes for that portion of her workout. If you're peaking for a big race or other event, plan to scale back on the length of your Cornerstone Workout in the final weeks before the race.

AUTUMN (OCTOBER THROUGH DECEMBER): TRANSITIONING

WEATHER FACTORS
Shorter days, changing weather patterns, cooler nights.

MOODS
A transition between the energy of the summer and the darkness of winter. A time for reflection, celebration, and transition.

OUTDOOR TRAINING OPPORTUNITIES
After the peak attained during the summer, autumn is a time to transition: allow a new level of fitness to settle into your body as you regroup, rest, and create new goals.

During autumn, you may wish to dial back your fitness efforts, adding a rest day or two as you allow your body to regroup and heal after the hard work of the summer. You will likely do a shorter endurance workout, and perhaps even a shorter Cornerstone Workout, depending on your overall energy level. Rest days are always advisable when you feel you need one. You may also choose to do some restorative work, such as yoga instead of running or other cardio. By adapting your twelve-week program with the idea of transition in mind, you will be able to find an activity level that gives you energy and allows you to rest when necessary.

TRAINING IN PHASES: ADAPT, BUILD, PEAK

The adventX program breaks each twelve-week fitness cycle into three phases, followed by a week of complete rest. Your twelve-week cycle will be made up of an Adaptation phase, a Building phase, and a Peaking phase. From there, you'll have a week of rest, the Transition phase (week thirteen). When you start to look at your workout year as one large cycle, you'll see that the phases match up very well to the seasons—an exciting and very organic way to train.

For your twelve weeks, we'll rely on a day-by-day program that illustrates this phased approach to training. These are simple, smart fitness concepts that anyone can learn and incorporate. I'm often reminded that the masters in any sport or practice are not good because of their volume of knowledge or experience, but because they have mastered a handful of basic moves or concepts extremely well.

By looking at any part of your training as a phase, you'll be able to set goals on a daily, weekly, monthly, and seasonal basis. We'll start by taking a closer look at how we can break each twelve-week seasonal training cycle into different phases; each specific phase is a time to focus on one or two big goals. This approach will also help you to avoid boredom and burnout, and keep your workouts fresh.

Weeks 1 to 3   **Adapting** to the new training program.

Weeks 4 to 7   **Building** strength and endurance.

Weeks 8 to 12   **Peaking** at a top level of performance.

Week 13 (rest) **Transitioning** after a time of peak effort.

This type of training is known as *periodization,* a concept introduced by the famed Canadian endocrinologist Dr. Hans Selye, whose groundbreaking work in the early twentieth century gave us a basic understanding of how stress affects our physiology. Later in the same century, physiologist Leo Matveyev and sports scientist Dr. Tudor Bompa expanded this work and changed the way we think about sports training. Through their work, we learned that by breaking up training seasons into separate periods or phases, you can maximize gains in performance and results, while avoiding overtraining, injury, working too hard, or burning out. In short, you are training like an athlete.

The following chart and explanations show what each of your twelve workout weeks will look like. For the program below, Phase 1 (Adapting) comprises Weeks 1 through 3; Phase 2 (Building) comprises Weeks 4 through 7; Phase 3 (Peaking) comprises Weeks 8 through 12; and the last phase is your week of rest, the Transitioning phase between twelve-week cycles.

Phase 1 consists of a day of cardiovascular endurance activity, a day of cross-training made up of the Daily Dozen and additional exercises, and a Cornerstone Workout (explained in detail later). You'll perform the Daily Dozen exercises each day of the week. The chart below illustrates one way to lay out your three main workouts and your Daily Dozen. Note that the Daily Dozen will be part of both your Cross-Training routine and your Cornerstone Workout; on the other five days, you can do your Daily Dozen anytime it's convenient.

PHASE 1   (ADAPTING)

DAY 1   Daily Dozen; Cardiovascular Endurance 20–60 minutes

DAY 2   Daily Dozen

DAY 3   Daily Dozen

DAY 4   Cross Train (Daily Dozen + 2 minutes activity between each exercise, such as jumping jacks, jump rope, light running)

DAY 5   Daily Dozen

DAY 6   Daily Dozen

DAY 7   Cornerstone Workout

In the second phase, you'll add two additional exercise sessions each week. These will be Circuit Training workouts, where you stay in motion for a pre-scribed amount of time while doing a succession of different exercises. You'll also have the choice to add a slightly longer cardiovascular endurance ses-sion. In addition, you'll have a few new choices for your cross-training day. You could do the same workout as in Phase 1 (weeks 1 to 3). You could also take one of the Cornerstone Workouts and simply cut it in half, so that you're working out for an hour or so. A third option is to make this day a Tempo Workout—a cardiovascular workout in which you spend a portion of the time working at a harder pace than you do in the longer cardiovascular endurance session. The chart below illustrates one way to fit the Phase 2 workouts into a workout week:

PHASE 2 (BUILDING)

DAY 1   Daily Dozen, Cardiovascular Endurance 45–120 minutes

DAY 2   Daily Dozen

DAY 3   Circuit Training (Daily Dozen + 5 minutes cardio warmup;
         3 times through the Basic Circuit; Home Stretch)

DAY 4   Cross Train (Daily Dozen + 2 minutes activity between each
         exercise, such as jumping jacks, jump rope, light running) or
         Tempo (10 minute warmup, 30–60 minutes cardio activity at
         70%–80% effort, 5–10-minute cooldown)

DAY 5   Circuit Training—same as Day 3

DAY 6   Daily Dozen

DAY 7   Cornerstone Workout

In Phase 3 (weeks 8 to 12), you'll sharpen your fitness and build to a peak. For your Circuit Training workout, you can use the same Basic Circuit you used in Phase 2, or feel free to substitute more advanced exercises in this circuit for a tougher workout. (At this phase of training, you'll be familiar with dozens of exercises, so you will have the information necessary to build a tougher circuit if you choose.) The significant difference from Phase 2 to Phase 3 is the intensity of your Cornerstone Workout—you'll definitely notice yourself getting stronger and the Cornerstone Workouts getting more challenging during this phase.

PHASE 3 (PEAKING)

DAY 1   Daily Dozen, Cardiovascular Endurance 45–180 minutes

DAY 2   Daily Dozen

DAY 3   Circuit Training (Daily Dozen + 5 minutes cardio warmup;
         3 times through the Basic Circuit; Home Stretch)

DAY 4   Cross Train (Daily Dozen + 2 minutes activity between each
         exercise, such as jumping jacks, jump rope, light running) or
         Tempo (10-minute warmup, 30–60 minutes cardio activity at
         70%–80% effort, 5–10-minute cooldown)

DAY 5   Circuit Training—same as Day 3

DAY 6   Daily Dozen

DAY 7   Cornerstone Workout

These weekly exercise charts may look a bit foreign right now, but don't worry: the goal is to introduce you to the flow of the entire twelve-week program and discuss the different types of workouts you'll embark on in this time. For each of the twelve chapters in Section 3, we'll discuss the full week of workouts in detail so that you can refer back to the book whenever you have a question.

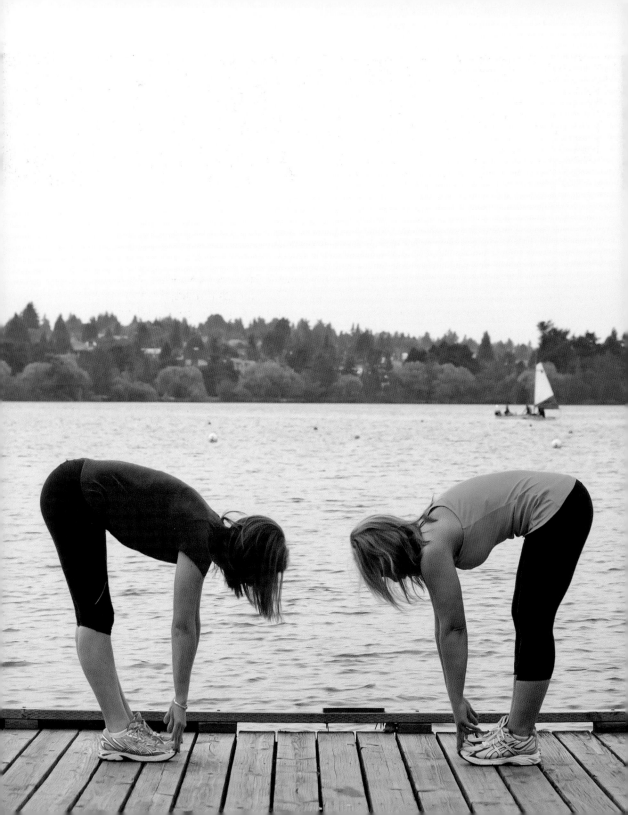

staying safe: injury prevention

With the abundance of vitamin D from the sun, the improved balance from walking and running on uneven terrain, and the gentleness of natural surfaces, you'll find that just getting outside for a workout will do quite a bit to improve your sense of health and well-being.

That said, it's impossible to guarantee that we'll always feel 100 percent healthy. There will always be colds, allergies, and potential injuries to contend with throughout our lives. However, the outdoor fitness lifestyle encourages making life choices that will give you the best possible chance to stay as healthy as possible. Exercise is a part of that, but there are equally important factors that have nothing to do with how many minutes it takes you to run a mile or how many push-ups you can do in a single set.

In this chapter, we'll talk about how to stay healthy, prevent injury, and rest appropriately to ensure that you're able to enjoy your outdoor workout program in the best of health.

BASIC SELF-CARE

These are steps we can all take to prepare for the healthiest possible outdoor fitness lifestyle:

- **A sensible progression in your fitness program**. (A rule of thumb is to increase intensity or volume of exercise by no more than 10 percent per week, as long as you are healthy and injury-free.)
- **Good nutrition**. (See the chapter "Fueling Your Journey" for more information on creating a healthy nutrition program.)

- **A balanced program that allows for restoration and relaxation**, in addition to periods of strength- and endurance-building exercise.
- **Proper clothing and footwear**.
- **An annual physical** with your doctor.

RESTORATION AND RELAXATION

To stay healthy and uninjured, I recommend incorporating some restoration and relaxation activities into your overall fitness program. These are some steps you can take to restore yourself between workouts:

- Massage
- Good nutrition, with a base of healthy, nutrient-dense foods
- Good hydration
- Relaxation: reading, watching a movie, napping
- Inspiring, motivating activities; spending time with friends and family; social events
- Meditation, breathing practice, and other relaxation techniques
- A daily walk, yoga, easy swim, or stretch

If there is one lesson we can take from nature, it is that everything should be in balance. While the animal kingdom possesses inherent intelligence about when to act and when to rest, humans tend to move too much, drive too much, sit too much, and do too much. Many of us have a hard time "switching off" and relaxing.

Restoration—literally, *restoring* yourself back to a fresh and rested state—is as important to your overall workout plan as any other aspect of this program. Training fatigues us. But we can restore the brightness and the tone of our bodies by resting. This process allows our bodies to repair themselves after the stress of workouts, and keeps us from becoming overtrained or injured. Remember a key equation: Training + Nutrition + Rest = Improvement.

Before you begin your twelve-week program, choose one day of the week to practice restoration. On this day, try to include a walk, or a period of stretching, yoga, or other relaxing movement for a period of time that allows you to relax. This could be for fifteen minutes or half an hour. Make it a habit, and it will play a large role in your fitness and health lifestyle. If you have trouble fitting in rest, remember the coaches' mantra: it's better to undertrain than overtrain. You can perform better when you're rested, even if you're slightly less fit than someone with more physical ability who has not taken time for rest and renewal.

STAYING SAFE OUTDOORS
There are very few conditions under which I wouldn't choose an outdoor workout. I find powerful weather to be exhilarating. I wouldn't recommend going kite-boarding in a hurricane, but I'll pull my collar up and my hat tight on a wild day and feel completely alive as the rain washes down my face and the wind buffets me around.

Staying warm and dry is the key to my enjoyment outdoors. Working out in rainy or cold weather requires the right gear to protect your body from the elements. This is one of the times when the saying, "There is no bad weather, only bad clothing," rings very true. If you make a mistake and get cold once in a while, it's okay; just be sure that you are not being reckless. Also, plan ahead so that you keep moving. Your body is a great natural heating system, but it shuts down the moment you stop exerting yourself, so a good strategy on cold days is to keep your breaks short and be sensible about your expectations. If you usually run three miles and you choose to tackle a ten-mile run for the first time on a cool day, how will you feel if you have to stop halfway and walk?

If you're going out alone, make sure to let someone know where you are going and when you expect to return. Also, be aware of dangerous conditions such as electrical storms or high winds, which can knock down tree branches.

PREVENTING HYPOTHERMIA
If you get both wet and cold, you risk hypothermia, where the core body temperature drops to 95 degrees Fahrenheit (35 degrees Celsius) or lower. Hypothermia is extremely dangerous. Constant shivering is the most obvious sign; others include confused thinking, clumsiness, slurred speech, or poor decision-making (such as trying to remove warm clothing). Remember that water is a far greater conductor of heat than air. You can comfortably sit in a 70-degree room, but if you were to be submerged in 70-degree water, you would develop hypothermia very quickly. Having solid workout clothing, including appropriate gear for rainy conditions, is a key part of training in the outdoors safely. And if you exhibit any signs of hypothermia, stop your workout immediately, go indoors, and get into dry, warm clothing as quickly as possible.

PREVENTING INJURY

When it comes to injury prevention, we can learn a lot from world-class athletes. Strength training is key, because one of the main jobs of muscles is to attenuate force. Should your muscles be insufficiently strong, that force will be directly absorbed by the joint, creating additional wear and tear that could easily lead to injury. Strength training, because it's so important, is built right into your Daily Dozen, Circuit Training, and Cornerstone Workouts.

Other activities you'll find top athletes engaging in to stay injury-free include icing sore muscles to reduce fatigue, and using a foam roller or other stretching devices (such as yoga blocks or bands) to stretch deeply. Ice baths are a favorite secret not only of elite athletes but many recreational athletes as well; a quick ice bath (three to five minutes) after a long endurance ride or run can go a long way to reduce muscle inflammation and increase the rate of the body's recovery after a hard effort.

WHAT TO DO WHEN YOU HURT

In the real world, many athletes will experience injuries, strains, or symptoms of overuse injuries. In this program, I challenge you to question the idea of "no pain, no gain." Pain is the body's way of telling us we have a problem. To push through pain can cause small problems to escalate into much larger ones.

Take time to learn a balanced approach to training and avoid the temptation to overdo it. Beware of listening to the prevailing attitude that you need to train until you drop. Consistent results are a product of consistent training. In other words, to finish *first*, we must first *finish*.

If you hurt, back off the intensity. This could be as simple as slowing down your exercise pace. From there, assess how you feel. If you start to feel better, then you're probably safe to continue your exercise for the day. However, if you experience a sharp pain in a joint or muscle, or any type of chest pain, shortness of breath, or faintness, do immediately stop and assess.

If you suffer any of the following during your workout, stop and seek medical attention immediately:

■ Swelling and/or unnatural heat or warmth around a joint. This can be a sign of infection.
■ Serious pain with movement of a limb.
■ Inability to bear weight on a limb.
■ Significant change in gait (an inability to walk normally).

COMMON INJURIES

These are some of the most common injuries to be aware of when you begin your training program. The recommended treatment plan for the injuries listed below is to consult with a doctor or a physical therapist. You may be familiar with the acronym RICE, which stands for **Rest, Ice, Compression,** and **Elevation**. These are all appropriate first-aid responses for the injuries described below. For more serious injuries, you may want to consult a specialist (see Sports Medicine Specialists, below).

ILIOTIBIAL (IT) BAND PAIN

The iliotibial band is a band of connective tissue that extends from the iliac crest (the bone on the side of your hip) down the outside of the thigh and across the knee joint, where it attaches to the tibia.

When the IT band gets tight and sore due to faulty biomechanics, especially in running and cycling, it can get very inflamed where it crosses the outside of the knee joint. This can create debilitating pain or a strong feeling of pronounced stiffness on the outside of the knee.

LOWER BACK PAIN

You'll know what this is because it will be impossible to ignore. Lower back pain has many causes. Often, mild low-back pain is helped by a well-designed exercise program, but if pain persists or worsens with any exercise, especially in conjunction with any leg pain or numbness (sciatica), this could indicate something more serious (for example, a lumbar disc or nerve injury).

ROTATOR CUFF (SHOULDER) PAIN

The rotator cuff is a set of muscles surrounding the shoulder joint that are responsible for the fine-tuning of its mechanics. Most commonly, injuries to the rotator cuff tendons will be caused by a fall on an outstretched arm or repeated overhead activities such as throwing. Frequently you will feel this pain when your arm goes above shoulder height during activities such as washing or brushing your hair, pulling off a t-shirt, or even reaching to get something from the back seat of the car.

With this condition in particular, pain is an important warning: exercises involving the shoulder joint should always be performed without pain. In this situation, pain may be an indication of imminent injury.

KNEE PAIN

There are many causes of knee pain. The most common form is discomfort around, behind, or below the kneecap. Frequent contributors to knee pain include inflexibility in the quadriceps muscles (front of the thigh), deconditioned hip muscles, and potentially faulty mechanics in the performance of common exercises like squats and lunges.

FOOT PAIN

Foot pain can be either transitory (such as muscle cramps and bruises) or a sign of a more serious condition such as a stress fracture or plantar fasciitis. Significant heel pain when taking your first steps out of bed in the morning could be an indicator of plantar fasciitis, an inflammation of the tendons on the underside of the foot, which requires an aggressive course of treatment. Any significant ongoing foot pain should be examined by a sports podiatrist or qualified physical therapist who can perform a full gait analysis and prescribe custom orthotics when necessary.

Your athletic shoes should fit well and be appropriate for the activity. Many athletic stores offer to analyze your gait and make recommendations based on your specific biomechanics. If you can take advantage of such a service, by all means do so.

ANKLE PAIN

Overpronation of the feet, where the foot rolls inward often because of a lack of arch support, can cause uneven strain on the ankle. In this type of situation, overpronation would likely overload the inside (medial) area of the joint.

Achilles tendon pain is common in athletes and can be a significant issue. Any ongoing palpable tenderness, especially if it includes chronic swelling in the tendon itself, should be examined by a doctor to discover the underlying source of the pain. You should not attempt to train through or ignore ankle pain.

SHIN PAIN

Shin splints (pain in the front of the shin) come in two varieties. *Anterior tibialis* pain occurs in the front of the lower leg, especially the outside of the tibia (the major bone of the lower leg), most often during a weight-bearing activity such as running. *Posterior* shin splints (sometimes referred to as medial shin splints) occur just inside or behind the tibia, and often derive from insufficient arch support or overpronation of the foot.

Common solutions include using proper footwear, strengthening the muscles of the foot and ankle, and using orthotics. One thing to consider when experiencing shin splints in particular is the progress of your training: if increased too aggressively, your foot and lower leg muscles may experience fatigue from work overload. We can't say it enough: progress at a slow enough pace so your body can adapt to the additional stress.

SPORTS MEDICINE SPECIALISTS

There are many medical specialists who can assist you in diagnosing and treating sports injuries. Below, we have included a list of specialists, along with their areas of expertise.

Medical doctor (MD): This could be your family doctor or an emergency room physician. Their job is to diagnose a medical problem and decide a treatment plan.

Physical therapist (PT): If you have a musculoskeletal injury, a physical therapist can prescribe a treatment plan to get you back in action. This may include instruction on proper biomechanics, stretching, or strengthening exercises.

Registered dietician (RD): A registered dietician has gone through four years of nutrition education. A board-certified specialist in sports dietetics (CSSD) can help you identify deficiencies in your nutrition program and design improvements to help increase strength, which will help to prevent injury.

Acupuncturist (LAC): Licensed acupuncturists work to ensure that the vital energy of your body circulates optimally. When other measures fail, it is often worthwhile to consider treating the problem with acupuncture.

Licensed massage practitioner (LMP): Many LMPs have specific training in sports-specific massage. Look for a practitioner who works with athletes.

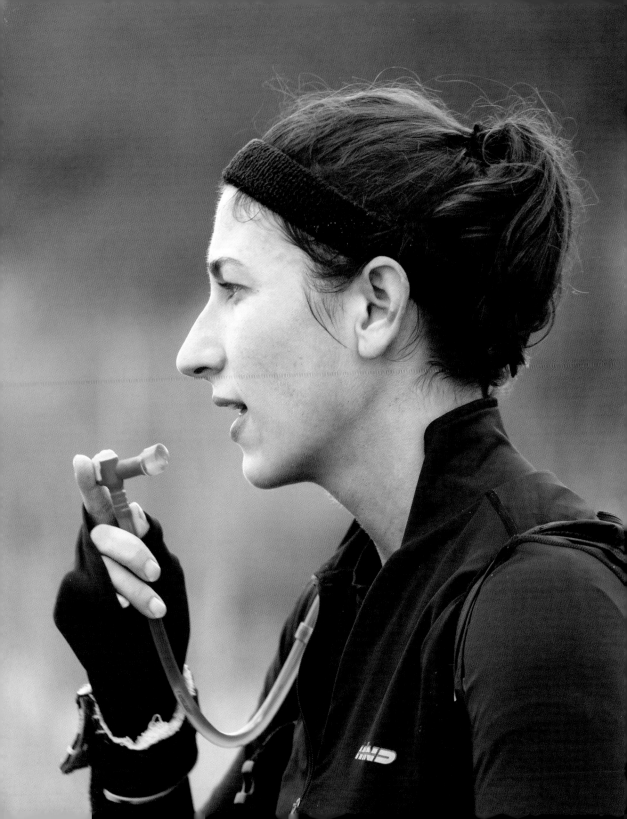

fueling
your journey

Nutrition is a science, not an opinion.

—Sally Hara, RD, CSSD, and adventX sports nutrition expert

As an outdoor athlete, my enthusiasm for nutrition has to do with understanding how best to provide my body with the nutrients that will enable me to feel good and to perform well. A huge advantage of training outdoors is that we're surrounded by the perfect balance of the natural world, and that extends to the way we balance what and how we eat. Athletic training conditions our bodies to use fuel efficiently.

Our national health crisis has shone the spotlight on nutrition in a way that is sometimes healthy, but often misleading. We are awash in information, yet good information is hard to find. Anyone can call themselves a nutritionist, and sometimes the nutritionist label is used to sell a product or supplement that may or may not be useful. I've learned that the demands on medical doctors are such that nutrition does not always top the priority list at medical schools. However, if your physician does diagnose or suspect a nutrition-related problem, he or she can refer you to a registered dietician. It takes at least four years to become an RD, including a clinical internship, and retaining the RD credential requires continuing education, which helps to ensure these professionals are current in their knowledge of the dynamic field of nutrition.

I highly recommend attending a talk or personal session with an RD who is a board-certified specialist in sports dietetics (CSSD) to objectively help you with the questions you may have about your nutrition and weight profile. An

RD can help you determine a healthy weight range for yourself, identify food sensitivities, suggest the right proportions of protein, carbohydrates, and fats in your diet, and help you put together a nutritional program that will sustain you for the long haul.

At adventX, we are lucky to have a registered dietician on our team. Sally Hara, MS, RD, CDE, CSSD, is a board-certified specialist in sports dietetics and the Pacific Northwest's leading authority on sports nutrition. She is also a cyclist and avid fitness enthusiast. In addition to her two degrees in nutrition science, she has a degree in exercise physiology.

Following is a question-and-answer session with Sally Hara that will address most of the questions you might have as you follow this program. In Appendix D, you will find additional references and resources on sports nutrition.

How much protein do I need?
Sally Hara: Most athletes require 1.2 to 1.4 grams of protein per kilogram of body weight (1 pound is equivalent to 2.2 kilograms). Ultra-endurance athletes may require up to 1.8 grams of protein per kilogram of body weight. This is typically not difficult for an athlete to get if he or she is eating a balanced, nutrient-dense diet and is responding appropriately to hunger cues. An ounce of meat, fish, poultry, or cheese contains about 7 grams of protein. Other good sources of protein are 1 to 2 tablespoons of nut butter, one egg, 1/4 cup cottage cheese, and 1/2 cup cooked legumes. A slice of bread, 1/3 cup of pasta or rice, or 1/2 cup cooked oatmeal can contain about 3 grams of protein each—check the nutritional label to be sure.

How much water should I drink?
SH: The general recommendation for daily fluid intake is about 64 to 80 ounces per day. This includes all fluids consumed, not just water. When you factor in endurance exercise, an athlete's fluid needs will increase. Although specific needs may vary depending on duration and intensity of the exercise, the ambient temperature and humidity, altitude, and individual differences between athletes, the following are general recommendations appropriate for most athletes.

2 to 3 hours before exercise	Drink about 20 oz. water or sports drink
During exercise	Drink 6 to 12 oz. every 15–20 minutes
After exercise	At least 20 oz. after exercise, with continued regular hydration for the remainder of the day. Ideally, enough to replace water lost via sweat, urine, and respiration. Consume 24 oz. for every pound of body weight lost during exercise.

Source: ADA. Position of the American Dietetic Association, Dietitians of Canada, and the American College of Sports Medicine: Nutrition and Athletic Performance, 2009

For serious endurance athletes, it may be worth the effort to calculate your sweat rate so that you can determine how much you need to drink during exercise to prevent dehydration. Use the formula in the following sidebar to determine your sweat rate.

How often should I eat?
SH: To optimize metabolism and both physiological and psychological performance (including mood, focus, and efficiency), I recommend eating every three to four hours. Serious athletes sometimes need to eat at least every two hours because of their high metabolism and energy needs. Spreading food intake throughout the day helps ensure that your brain and body will have enough energy to function properly during the day. Eating at regular intervals helps prevent overeating at the end of the day caused by extreme hunger. It seems paradoxical, but eating frequently can actually help regulate body weight better than skipping meals and snacks. If a person is in tune with their natural hunger and fullness signals, the best advice is simply to eat when you're hungry and stop when you're satisfied. Unfortunately, people who have a history of dieting often are disconnected from these signals because they have a history of ignoring them. If you are truly hungry, eat high-quality, nutrient-dense food. Hunger is a signal that your body is asking for more energy. Just respond to hunger with the most nutrient-dense food available.

determining sweat rate

While there's no need to train like an elite athlete most of the time, one place where it may be helpful is when you're just beginning to learn how much fluid your body needs during a period of long endurance activity. Here's a basic formula that can help you determine how much to drink during endurance exercise.

First, weigh yourself before you begin a long workout (such as a two-hour Cornerstone Workout). Carry a measured amount of fluid (water or sports drink) with you and note how much you drink during your workout. After the workout, weigh yourself again. Now, plug those numbers into the following equation:

A=(pre-exercise body weight in pounds) – (post-exercise body weight in pounds)– (ounces of fluid consumed divided by 16), B =Exercise time in hours. *Your sweat rate per hour will be A divided by B.*

For example, a 150-pound man who weighs 148 pounds after a two-hour run during which he consumed 16 ounces (or one pound) of a sports drink would have a sweat rate of: A =(150 pounds pre-exercise weight)– (148 pounds post-exercise weight)–1 (16 ounces divided by 16) = 1, B = 2. *A divided by B = 1/2 pound, or 8 ounces per hour.* Therefore, this athlete would do well to consider consuming an additional 8 ounces of fluid for every hour of endurance exercise.

What do you mean when you refer to certain foods as "nutrient dense"?
SH: Nutrient density is a measure of the nutrients in a food relative to the energy (calories) it provides. If a food has more nutrients and fewer calories, it's considered nutrient dense: you are getting a lot of bang for your buck. The following chart illustrates how two foods with the same energy (calorie) content can vary significantly in nutrient density. The banana is clearly more nutrient dense than the low-calorie cookie. The message is simple: not all calories are created equal.

	Banana	Chocolate Chip Cookie 100-calorie pack
Amount Per Serving	*1 medium*	*1 package*
Calories	105	100
Fat	0.39 g	3 g
Sodium	1.2 mg	140 mg
Potassium	422 mg	0 mg
Carbohydrate	27 g	18 g
Dietary Fiber	3 g	1 g
Protein	1 g	1 g
Vitamin A	2%	0%
Calcium	1%	0%
Thiamin	2%	0%
Niacin	4%	0%
Vitamin B6	22%	0%
Phosphorus	3%	0%
Selenium	2%	0%
Vitamin C	17%	0%
Iron	2%	4%
Riboflavin	5%	0%
Manganese	16%	0%
Copper	5%	0%

How do I know when I'm getting the correct mix of macronutrients (carbohy-drates, proteins, and fat) to enable my best performance?

SH: This is one issue a sports dietician can help you determine. Most ath-letes think they need much more protein than they actually do, and many vastly underestimate their need for carbohydrates. While protein is necessary to build and repair muscles and other tissues, carbohydrate is the preferred fuel for exercise (even for strength training). Protein is building material, car-bohydrates are fuel. The more you work out, the more fuel you need.

Do I have to eat breakfast?

SH: For optimal health and performance, yes. When we wake up in the morning, our glycogen stores are significantly depleted, because that is our primary energy source when we sleep.

What do you eat before a morning training session?

SH: Usually a light but balanced meal or snack is best; something that con-tains mostly carbohydrate and a little protein for longer workouts is ideal. The size of the meal depends on the duration and intensity of the workout. Yogurt with granola or fruit can work well. Including a combination of simple and complex carbohydrates provides both an immediate energy source (simple carbs) and one that is digested more slowly, giving you more energy over time (complex carbs). An example of a meal that serves this purpose could be oatmeal with soymilk and raisins.

How much should I eat before training?

SH: This depends on how long it has been since you've eaten, what you last ate, and the type, duration, and intensity of your workout. As an example, for a two-hour Cornerstone Workout done first thing in the morning before your first meal of the day, you may want to eat 200 to 300 calories of mostly carbohydrates, like a fiber-rich cereal. Do this an hour before starting, and have an energy gel or other snack of around 100 calories one hour into the workout. Every body is different; experiment to see what works best for you.

How can I determine how many calories I need to consume?

SH: Many variables determine energy needs, including age, gender, height, weight, body composition, and the fitness level of the athlete, as well as the type, intensity, and duration of the exercise. Energy needs may be estimated by formulas that include these variables (metabolic calculations). Similar formulas using heart rate to estimate intensity are available (some are even programmed into heart rate monitors). These formulas all begin with estimating your basal metabolic rate (BMR). The formula thought to be most accurate for this is the Mifflin–St. Jeor equation (see sidebar on next page). There are a few online resources that can do this calculation for you as well. The BMR essentially represents the amount of energy you need to keep your body running if you never got out of bed in the morning. Once you even sit up, your energy needs increase. For this reason the BMR must be multiplied by an activity factor to estimate daily maintenance needs. Many sites will list this activity factor in terms of activity level (sedentary, active, very active, etc.). This can give a fairly good estimate of energy expenditure, up to a point. For a more accurate number, BMR can also be measured if you have access to the necessary equipment (often exercise physiologists or sports medicine clinics will have these types of machines).

Should I eat before a workout? What can I eat and how soon before the workout?
SH: Yes. I recommend a snack with carbohydrates (fruit, granola bar, smoothie, etc.) within two hours prior to exercise. If you will be training for over ninety minutes, it is also good to include a protein source (peanut butter, yogurt, meat, soy products, etc.) to help stabilize your blood sugar for a longer period of time. How close to your workout you eat depends on you. Some people can eat a three-course meal five minutes before intense exercise, while others can barely tolerate a small yogurt two hours before the workout. This is very individual.

What should I eat after a workout and how soon after?
SH: The most important requirements for recovery are carbohydrates, fluids, and electrolytes. The perfect recovery snack is chocolate milk—it offers all of this plus a little protein. There are other options, of course, but the focus should be on carbs and hydration. A small amount of protein may also be helpful for post-exercise recovery, but the bulk of your post-exercise meal should be made up of carbohydrates. Remember to eat something within one hour after exercise to get a jump on replenishing your glycogen stores.

calculating basal metabolic rate (BMR)

The Mifflin–St. Jeor equation, shown below, can be used to calculate your approximate BMR.

Men: BMR = [10 x body weight in kilograms] + [6.25 x height in centimeters] -
[5 x age in years] + 5

Women: BMR = [10 x body weight in kilograms] + [6.25 x height in centimeters] -
[5 x age in years] - 161

Should I take a multivitamin?

SH: In theory, we should be able to get all of our vitamins and minerals from the food we eat. Even if there is a slightly higher nutritional need in endurance athletes, the increased amount of food necessary to meet energy demands should contain the additional vitamins and minerals needed as well. That said, not everyone has a perfect diet, so a basic multivitamin may not be a bad idea. There is no need to overspend on specialized vitamins, however. For instance, those little packets with four to six vitamin pills in them are mostly a marketing ploy.

I don't eat fish—should I take fish oil supplements?

SH: Fish oil supplements are an excellent idea. The omega-3 fatty acids in these supplements have multiple documented benefits, including cholesterol balance, anti-inflammatory effects, and mood stabilization. A good substitute for vegetarians would be flaxseed oil.

What type of beverage should go into my water bottle when I'm exercising—something with electrolytes?

SH: For anyone exercising over sixty minutes, I recommend a sports drink containing both electrolytes and carbohydrates. Since you should be fueling as you go, this is a convenient way to take in the recommended carbohydrates.

Alternatively, you could fill the bottle with an electrolyte-only drink and eat solid foods as an energy source. It really depends on the sport and whether or not you typically eat while training. Either way, fluids and electrolytes are both important to have in your sports bottle.

How does alcohol affect my performance?
SH: It's all about timing and moderation. Alcohol is a known diuretic and can lead to significant dehydration and electrolyte imbalances. If you have an occasional beer, rehydrate before turning in for the night and limit yourself to one to two drinks per day. Alcohol is a known toxin that can hinder liver functions, including the ability of the liver to produce blood sugar from glycogen (for fuel) during exercise.

How much fiber do I need?
SH: The current recommendation is about 30 grams of fiber per day. Consuming whole grains most of the time and getting at least five servings of fruits and vegetables a day will likely provide this amount of fiber easily.

What if I don't have much time to cook?
SH: This is a big problem in our society. Some strategies could include cooking once a week and freezing several meals that you can easily heat up later. One great tool for athletes is a slow cooker. You can chop meat, vegetables, and spices, put them in a slow cooker for eight hours, and you'll have wonderful meals. Personally I enjoy curries, chili, stews, soups, and even baked potatoes. It's easy, safe (you can leave it on all day), inexpensive ($50 to $100), and the cooking method does not leach vitamins or minerals, nor does it destroy nutrients with excessive heat.

For vegetarians, are there specific things to know about eating for athletic performance?
SH: The basic needs for vegetarian athletes are the same as for other athletes. What differs is the source of some of the nutrients (especially protein, iron, B12, and calcium). A great resource for this is the book *The Vegetarian's Sports Nutrition Guide*, by Lisa Dorfman, RD, CSSD (see Appendix D).

Vegetarians should pay particular attention to getting enough protein, but it's not that difficult to do. The main sources of protein for vegetarians are legumes (such as dried beans, peas, and lentils), soy products, and (for nonvegans) milk, cheese, yogurt, and eggs. The good thing about vegetarian protein sources is that most also contain carbohydrates, which are an athlete's best friend.

Iron, one of the nutrients that all vegetarians must be aware of, is found abundantly in animal products but sparsely in plant products. Some good sources of iron for vegetarians include dried beans and dark green leafy vegetables. Iron absorption is increased by eating foods containing vitamin C together with iron-rich foods in the same meal.

If I am a vegetarian, how can I get enough vitamin B12?
SH: Vitamin B12 is found only in animal products. Lacto-ovo vegetarians can get B12 from dairy products and eggs. Vegans (who eat only plant products) need to supplement their diet with B12 either by including nutritional yeast, foods that have been fortified with it (like some soy milks), or by taking a B12 supplement. The recommended intake of B12 for adults is 2.4 micrograms daily. Inadequate B12 can result in a condition called *macrocytic anemia*, in which you will be overly tired and have difficulty training and recovering from exercise.

How do I know if I'm getting enough iron?
SH: Iron deficiencies are common in endurance athletes, especially runners. There is controversy over why this occurs. Iron plays a key role in transporting oxygen to the muscles. This increases the need for iron in endurance athletes. Athletes who overtrain will often develop iron-deficiency anemia despite consuming what should be adequate iron, because a body that is in a stressed state from overtraining makes the iron unavailable. If you have a history of iron deficiency (determined by simple blood tests your doctor can order), taking an iron supplement routinely is a good idea. If this doesn't fix the problem, you may need to examine your training and nutrition habits. Certainly, making sure to include iron-rich foods (especially red meat, which is very high in iron) is very important.

What is carbohydrate loading? When do I need to carbo-load for an endurance event?
SH: Carbohydrate loading is essentially a means of increasing muscle glycogen stores. It has been shown to greatly improve athletic performance in events lasting 90 to 120 minutes or longer. An athlete using carbohydrate

loading can double muscle glycogen stores and thus spare glycogen during the event. There are protocols that can be very helpful to accomplish this, but carbohydrate loading takes about a week to do right; it's more than consuming a big pasta dinner the night before an event. Consult a sports dietician for more information on carbo-loading protocols if you're preparing for a long distance event, such as a marathon or a long triathlon.

In summary, nutrition for optimal sports performance is a science and an art. It should be just as much a part of your training as your workouts, your rest, and your recovery. Like investing in a good pair of shoes, professional bike fit, quality climbing gear, or a skilled coach, investing in a professional sports nutrition consultation is well worth the cost, and will continue to pay off for years to come.

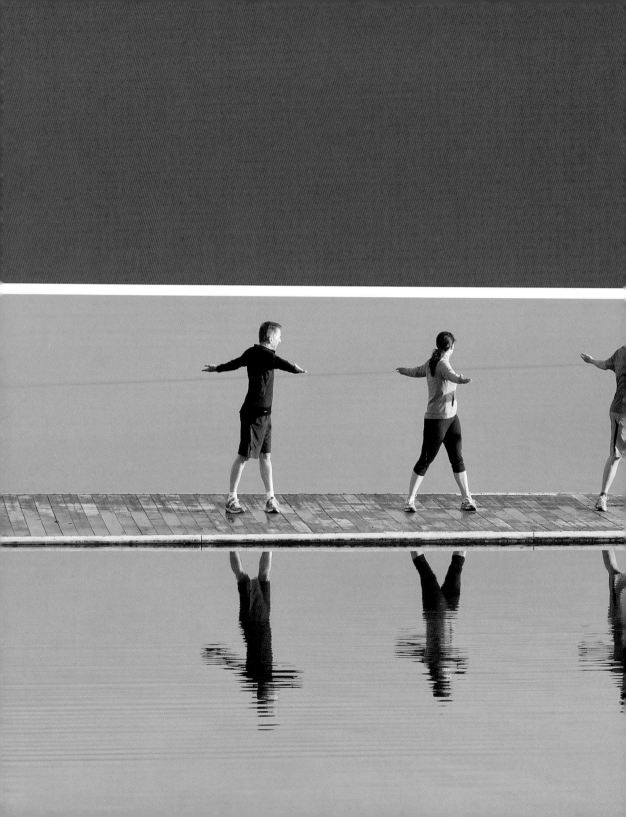

get set

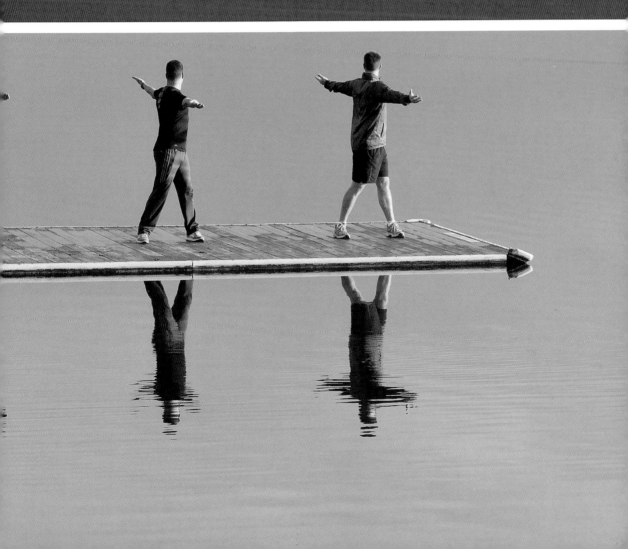

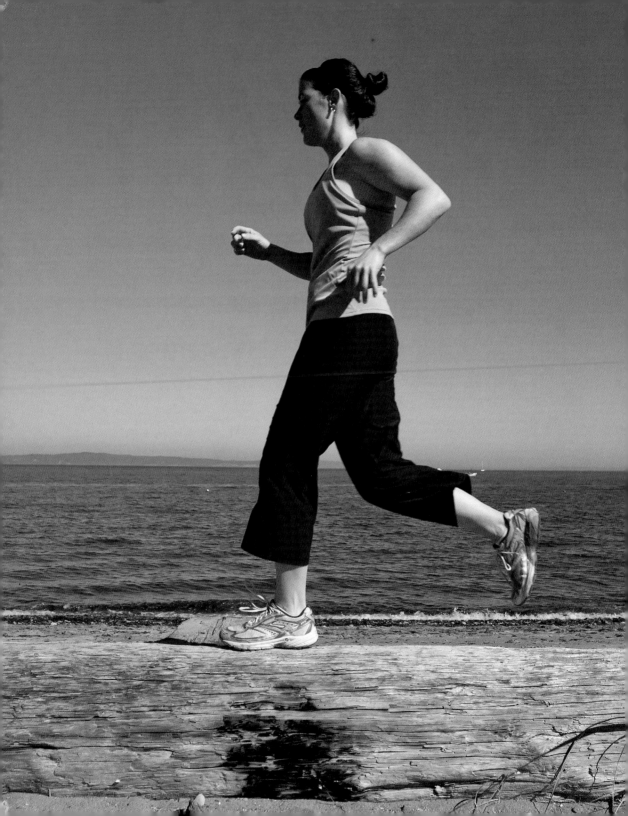

preparation

A little advance preparation will go a long way as you begin your outdoor fitness program. The following sections deal with some of the most important things to consider when readying yourself for your program: a gear list, suggested workout attire by season and type of weather, and tips for setting aside the time for your workouts.

GEAR

The following list of suggested gear items can all be purchased at a sporting goods store.

- A sports watch with a stopwatch feature. You'll use this to time each segment of your workout and to note the time it takes you to perform your fitness tests.
- A water bottle or a hydration system such as a CamelBak, able to carry about 1 liter of water that you can sip throughout your workout.
- Energy snack: an easily digestible snack of around 200 calories that you can eat halfway through your Cornerstone Workout if you need it. A sports bar or energy gel is perfect.
- A small notepad and pen, to record the results of timed runs and other information.
- A small first-aid kit including adhesive bandages, a topical ointment, and an elastic or compression bandage to treat minor injuries.
- A cell phone, especially if you're exercising alone.
- Sunscreen and sunglasses for sunny days (even in the winter).

- A 20-yard cord or thin rope with a 10-yard mark measured on it for several of the drills in the Cornerstone Workouts.
- (Optional) A small waist pack to carry your phone, energy snack, sunscreen, etc.
- (Optional) Ten small plastic orange cones to mark workout stations during your Circuit Training sessions.
- (Optional) A jump rope.
- (Optional) A resistance band.

WORKOUT ATTIRE BY THE SEASON

Our motto is simple: Dress for success. No one has ever dissolved in one of our rainy-day classes. Depending on your location and the time of year, we may experience more "exciting" weather such as rain or wind. Nature offers a full spectrum of extremes, and we can do many things to be comfortable in just about all conditions while experiencing the beauty and variety of diverse weather situations.

Clothing will be determined by several factors, including weather (temperature, level of precipitation, sun), wind chill factor (if any), length of time you will be outdoors, terrain, and intensity of training. The key is *layering*—making sure you have enough protection against the elements while providing yourself with several choices of attire.

Some of the exercises in this program may be performed on the ground. When it's dry, this won't present a problem, but your outdoor workout clothes may get a bit dirty at times, so plan ahead. Some athletes like a separate layer just to put on the ground, but this isn't essential; it's your call, depending on your comfort level.

THE KEY TO LAYERING: EVAPORATION, INSULATION, AND PROTECTION

I like to categorize outdoor fitness clothing by placing each item into one of three main layers.

Evaporation
Evaporation layers are thin, synthetic-based materials that "wick" or transport

moisture away from the skin. Unlike cotton, which absorbs moisture, synthetic (or "technical") apparel is constructed from synthetic fibers that, through the weight and weave of the material, allow moisture and heat to pass through the fabric. This is important because water conducts heat much faster than dry air. The result is that your sweat-soaked cotton garment is actually stealing your body heat on a cold day, possibly leading to hypothermia, and trapping the moisture on a hot day, preventing cooling and possibly leading to heat exhaustion or even heat stroke.

Consider the following for your evaporation layer:

- A technical fabric t-shirt
- Running shorts or capris
- Sports socks with wicking capability
- Light baseball hat (for sunny days)
- A technical fabric sports bra (for women)

Insulation

Insulation layers for the outdoor fitness enthusiast consist mainly of clothing that you might use before or after your workout. Given the moderate to high intensity of your workouts, you won't need much in the way of insulation, as you will create sufficient heat as you train. But you may feel chilled soon after completing your workout, so have an insulation layer on hand. An exception would be a cold climate where temperatures regularly drop below freezing, or when you're training in the early morning and at night. In these conditions, a light or midweight fleece layer can be useful during the workout itself.

For pants, consider a pair of nylon pants (some outdoor retailers sell nylon pants that zip off at the knees to double as shorts). For your upper body, consider the following for your insulation layer, in order from lightest to heaviest:

- A light nylon jacket
- A long-sleeve lightweight wool top
- A soft-shell sports jacket
- A fleece jacket

Protection

A protective layer keeps you from being adversely affected by elements such as rain, snow, and wind. This is normally a synthetic layer: it could be a nylon jacket or a technical piece constructed from Gore-Tex or a similar waterproof fabric. "Breathable" materials are constructed of layers, including a membrane that acts like the skin as it breathes, to transport heat and moisture away from the body while protecting against wind and rain. For your longer Cornerstone Workouts, a lighter garment usually works better than a heavy one.

Consider the following for your protection layer:

- A nylon windbreaker
- A light, waterproof jacket (Gore-Tex or similar material)

Additional Layers and Accessories

Protecting yourself isn't just a matter of having the best jacket and pants; you also want to protect your extremities. For head and hands, putting on (or taking off) a light wool hat or gloves can be the fastest way to adjust your comfort level. You can stow them in a pocket or a small backpack when you're not using them. As with clothing, dress for the occasion and remember that, generally speaking for these workouts, "lighter is right(er)."

FOOTWEAR

Ensure that your shoes allow you to move around without discomfort. If you have access to an athletic shoe store where the staff can recommend shoes for your foot shape and gait, that will be your best bet. This is one area where having a professional assessment will pay off greatly. The right shoe will protect your feet from injury and should offer protection from the elements.

SUN AND WIND PROTECTION

Don't forget sunscreen and lip protection for sun, cold, and wind. Moisturizing creams with SPF provide a layer of protection, as does SPF-enhanced lip balm. Protect your eyes as well—sunglasses guard against bright sunshine, plus dust, debris, and even the stray insect that gets in your airspace.

MAKE OUTDOOR EXERCISE PART OF YOUR LIFESTYLE

Preparation will make everything easier. Once your clothing is assembled, reserve a slot of time in your calendar just for your workouts.

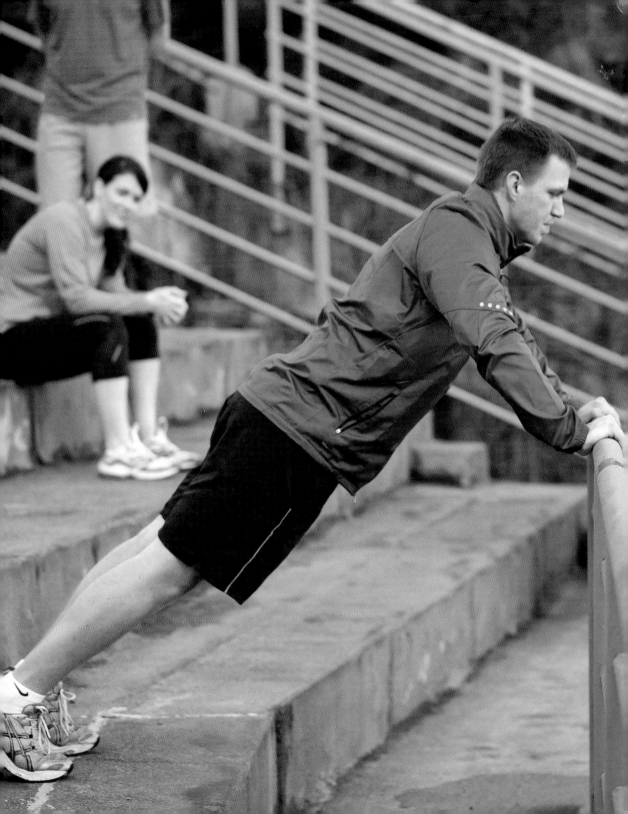

If you don't have time for a particular workout on a particular day, just do as much of it as you have time for, making sure to take a quick pass through the Home Stretch afterward. The important thing is moderation and consistency. All of the times listed in this book for workouts are approximate, not hard-and-fast rules.

Plan out your days so that you know when and where you'll work out. Perhaps first thing in the morning is best for you; in that case, you'll want to set out your gear and pack your bag the night before. If the afternoons or evenings work better, ensure success by bringing your gear to work (if you're working out after a workday) or setting it in a prominent place at home.

CHALLENGE BY CHOICE: SETTING GOALS

"What would you do if you knew you could not fail?" Honestly answered, that question can provide the motivation to start on a journey of limitless gain, growth, and personal accomplishment. We often have difficulty grasping how much we are capable of accomplishing, yet we may be criticized by others who think our goals are too far-reaching. Ordinary people do extraordinary things all the time. If your goals feel unrealistic, they may be too small, not too big—and small goals can fail to motivate us. Are we really going to roll out of bed each day and train for a small result? I urge you to choose goals that make you feel excited and empowered. Powerful feelings help us train better, perform better, and improve our overall results.

What would you do *if you knew you could not fail?* Would you want to lose a few pounds? Or would you like to summit a 14,000-foot mountain? Can you sense the difference in energy between those goals? You might lose those pounds training for a mountain climb—but your focus will be on something so much bigger than yourself and more attuned to the natural world, inspiring you to make a commitment to yourself and your fitness that you may only now sense building inside.

As you move forward in your workout program, you might find that you're inspired by other goals. All goals are valid, whether it's simply a goal to feel healthier and stronger and to set aside two hours a week to enjoy an outdoor exercise session, or to try for a personal goal such as summiting a mountain, doing your first triathlon, or setting a lifetime personal best in a race or other activity. Many adventX athletes take the confidence they've gotten from this program to accomplish major career goals, recover from serious health issues, and build lives of true contentment and happiness.

THE GOAL-SETTING PROCESS

Start by completing the **adventX On-Target Questionnaire** in Appendix C of this book. As you complete this questionnaire, remember that it may take longer than one twelve-week program to achieve some of your goals—and for a lifelong goal, it *should* take longer than that. Lifelong goals should capture your imagination, enliven your spirit, and make every day worth living. Hold on to that image as you work through the questionnaire to map out your own goals for the next twelve weeks.

CREATE YOUR OUTDOOR WORKOUT SPACE

The concept of exercise being separate from the rest of our lives is very modern. For millennia, exercise was a necessary component of survival and growth, whereas today we have to make time for exercise. Whether it's for health or recreation, competition or enjoyment, we usually go to a gym to work out, and then go back outside, plop into our cars, and drive off to the rest of our lives. A big part of this book is considering the possibility that **there is no gym separate from the rest of your life**. The picnic table in the park across the street, or stairs connecting two streets to one another in a big city could be the best pieces of exercise equipment you'll ever use. If water inspires you, your gym could be the shore of a local lake or river. If great expanses of grass get you going, a large park could be your best bet. Think of it this way: *we live in our gym*. Explore your own community to find a suitable outdoor space for your workouts. Go to a place you would enjoy exercising and take inventory of the opportunities you find there. Look for any of the following features in your outdoor workout space:

▪ Surfaces: a baseball field, soccer field, or other green space; sand (a beach or sand pit); paved paths.
▪ Features: picnic tables, park benches, stairs.
▪ Natural environment: trees (for shade and wind protection), logs, hills, flat spaces.
▪ Views: overlooks or other scenery (a view of a lake, river, or mountains can be particularly inspiring when working out).

- Ease of access: can you get to it easily by walking, biking, or taking the bus? Would you have to drive there?
- Impact on others: is it a busy trail or open space? You may wish to use open spaces to avoid affecting others' enjoyment of the park.

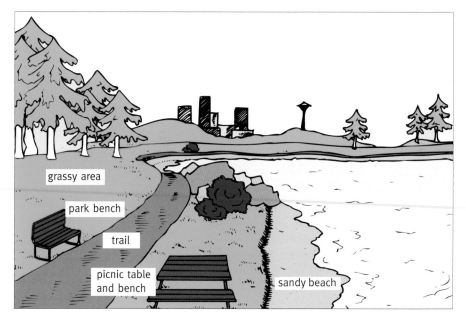

An ideal outdoor gym

the basic workouts

This chapter provides an overview of the two basic sets of movements you'll use throughout this program: the Daily Dozen and the Home Stretch. The Daily Dozen is a set of twelve simple exercises you can do anywhere, anytime, that encompass flexibility, strength, and endurance. The Home Stretch is your regular stretching routine. Do this whenever you feel you need extra flexibility, and especially after your regular workouts to prevent muscle tightness and fatigue.

THE DAILY DOZEN: CALISTHENICS FOR EVERYDAY CONDITIONING

I recommend you perform the Daily Dozen every day. You need no equipment, not even workout clothing—you can even do this workout in your pajamas. Each exercise takes 1 minute (45 seconds of movement followed by 15 seconds of rest), so the entire routine will take just 12 minutes a day. If you think about it, those 12 minutes each day add up to 18 hours in 90 days. That's a huge amount of strengthening and fitness to gain by doing something in the time it takes to brew coffee in the morning.

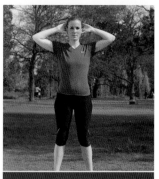

steam engine (1)

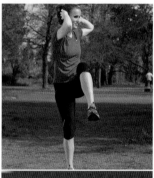

steam engine (2)

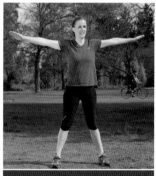

toe toucher (1)

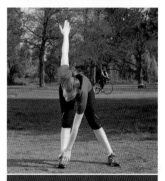

toe toucher (2)

STEAM ENGINE

How to do it: Stand with your feet shoulder width apart and your hands clasped behind your head. Lift your left knee, simultaneously bending and twisting to touch your right elbow to the left knee, keeping the muscles of your core (your abdominals and lower back) engaged. Alternate, using your right knee and left elbow, keeping your hands behind your head.

Notes: This great compound exercise stretches the hamstrings and back muscles in several directions: up, down, and diagonal. It also promotes good balance: when the knee comes up, you're balancing on the standing leg. And it's a good exercise for your core muscles: start with good posture and stomach muscles tight through the full range of motion to exercise your lower back, abdominal, and chest muscles.

TOE TOUCHER

How to do it: Stand with your feet hip width apart and arms extended straight out to your sides at a 90-degree angle from your body. Bend from the waist as you touch your left hand to your right foot, return to standing position, and then bend again to touch your right hand to your left foot. Alternate sides, keeping your arms straight at all times. The movement here comes from the waist. Keep your core muscles engaged and your back straight (don't hunch over).

Notes: This is a forward bend with a slight twist, which exercises the abdominal muscles, lower core muscles, hamstrings, and glutes. In the morning, it can be tough if the legs are tight—go gently, taking care to warm up. Don't press to go all the way down to your feet if you're feeling tight.

TWISTER

How to do it: Start in the same posture as the Toe Toucher. Slowly twist at the waist to the left as far as you can, and then slowly return to facing front, before twisting to the right. The motion here comes from the hips, not your back, as you twist side to side. The head moves in the direction of the twist, along with the arms. As with all of these exercises, keep your core engaged. **Notes:** Pause at the end of each twist before moving in the opposite direction. Take care not to throw your body around on this movement. Go through the full range of motion for your core muscles (abdominals and lower back). Practice care when performing this movement if you have any underlying lower-back problems, going slowly through the full range, and stop if you have any pain in your back.

SIDE BENDER

How to do it: Stand with your feet together, arms raised straight above your head, palms facing together. Keeping your arms straight, slowly bend to the right. Slowly straighten and bend to the left. Alternate sides. **Notes:** This exercise works the sides of your abdominal muscles (called the obliques). Stand as tall as you can with your hands to the sky, palms together. Remember that the motion is side to side—not forward, and not twisting. Imagine that your body is sandwiched between two panes of glass and all you can do is move side to side. As with the Twister, be mindful of your lower back, holding your abdominal core tight, stopping if you feel discomfort.

THREE-QUARTER SQUAT

How to do it: Stand with legs shoulder width apart and arms at your sides. Swing your arms forward and up, raising them above your head, palms facing forward. At the same time, bend your knees as if you were sitting in a chair. Hold the Squat briefly, then stand up by pushing through your heels, until you are in a full upright standing position.

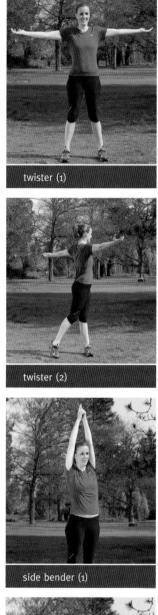

twister (1)

twister (2)

side bender (1)

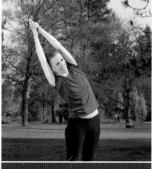

side bender (2)

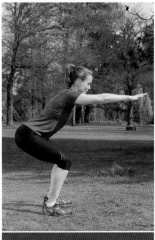

three-quarter squat

Notes: Many people refer to the Squat as the king of exercises because it's an all-body exercise that works everything from the feet to the fingertips when performed correctly. It also contributes to good balance—especially important as you get older. Keep it simple: stand upright with good posture, feet shoulder distance apart with your weight on your heels. Imagine roots underneath your heels, anchoring you to the ground. Keep your stomach muscles tight. Then think of sending your hips backward to achieve a sitting movement, as though you're easing into a chair. As you rise, drive the weight of your body into your heels until you are fully upright. Be sure to keep your back straight at all times. If you feel your back curving, you've probably gone a little too far. If you can't go down very far, that's okay; it's better to do a small Squat, keeping good form, than a deep Squat that causes you to bend your back.

LUNGE

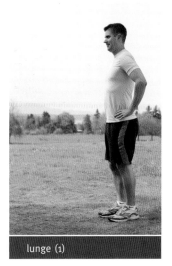

lunge (1)

How to do it: Stand upright, feet and legs together, hands on hips, elbows out to sides. Step your right leg backward. Bend your left knee until the kneecap is directly above your foot, causing the leg to form a 90-degree angle. Simultaneously lower your right leg until the knee almost rests on the ground, forming another 90-degree angle. Step back to starting position, and repeat, stepping backward with the left leg. Continue to alternate legs.

Notes: Lunges are a simple exercise as long as you maintain good posture. When you step backward, make sure you're not stepping too far or too little. On the downward position on the Lunge, the forward knee should be just over the forward ankle. Technically, the correct angle for the shin bone is a bit more than 90 degrees, but it's important not to let the knee travel out too far over the ankle. The motion of the leg as you move into the Lunge should be downward, not forward. If, after the initial step backward, your front knee moves forward instead

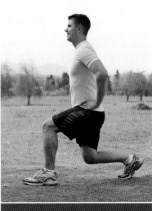

lunge (2)

of down, you're compromising your knee. Another tip is to make sure that the knee on the forward leg is in line with the hip on the same side of the body—it should not push to the left or to the right. If the movement challenges you at first, try taking a smaller step backward, or lower your back knee less.

SUMO SQUAT

How to do it: Stand with your feet a little wider than hip distance apart, toes pointing out at 45-degree angles. Put your hands on your hips and bend your knees out to the sides, making sure to keep them in line with the toes. Lower your body in a Squat until your thighs are parallel to the ground, and then push up through your heels to a standing position. Repeat.

Notes: With the hips more open than in the Three-Quarter Squat, this exercise allows you to go deeper into the movement. The same rules apply as in a regular Squat: keep your weight on your heels, and keep your abdominals, glutes, and hamstrings tight and strong as you move through the exercise. You can reach up to the sky with your arms as you move down into the Squat, exercising the chest and the upper back.

PUSH-UP

How to do it: Start with palms and toes on the ground, body in the air, as straight and strong as possible. Your arms should be directly underneath your shoulders, and you can spread your fingers wide for stability. (If this is more of a challenge than you'd like right now, do a modified Push-up with your knees on the ground.) Keeping the back and neck straight, inhale, bend your elbows and lower yourself until you are about 2 inches off the ground. Exhale as you push back up into the starting position. Repeat.

Notes: Push-ups are a major, full-body exercise. The most important part of the Push-up is the position in which you begin the movement. Imagine a plank of

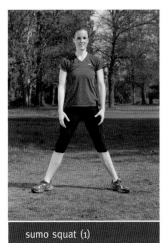
sumo squat (1)

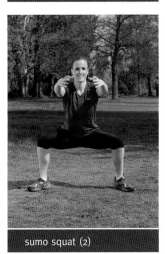
sumo squat (2)

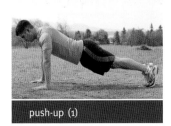
push-up (1)

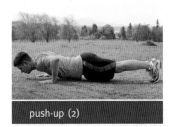
push-up (2)

the push-up

Push-ups are one of those exercises with a *reputation:* many people find them very intimidating. At adventX, we simply modify the exercise as needed to work with the upper-body strength of each athlete, with the expectation that each athlete will eventually be able to perform many push-ups, no matter what their starting strength was. If full push-ups are hard at first, definitely use the knees-to-ground variation, but consider that by changing your mind-set, you might just surprise yourself. Just practice, work within your effort level, and pretty soon you'll be amazed at what you can do.

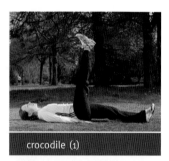
crocodile (1)

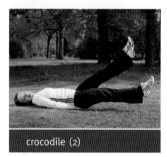
crocodile (2)

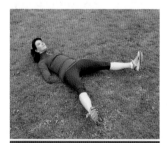
scissors (1)

wood on your back to keep good alignment through-out. Your hands should be shoulder width apart, fingers pointing forward. Breathing is especially important for the Push-up; remember to inhale on the downward phase of the movement, and exhale on the upward phase. As you push up, be aware of pulling your elbows into your body, and remember to engage all of your core muscles (abdominals and lower back).

CROCODILE

How to do it: Lie on the ground on your back with legs extended, and place your hands under your buttocks. Your head and neck should be slightly off the ground, eyes looking up to the sky. Lift both legs just off the ground using your abdominal muscles. Keeping your left leg in place, raise your right leg straight up to a 90-degree angle from your body. Lower the right to just above the ground while at the same time raising the left straight up. Continue alternating legs.

SCISSORS

How to do it: Start in the same position as in the Crocodile, above. Move the legs apart as far as you can, an inch or so off the ground, and then slowly move them together, crossing your right leg over your left (if you can). Extend the legs apart again, and then move them together, this time crossing left leg over right. Repeat. **Notes:** Both Crocodiles and Scissors are advanced exercises. They are great strengtheners, but can also put some pressure on the lower back, so take care if you have any lower back issues—slow down and go through the full range of motion, never pushing through pain. Beginners would do well to bend their knees slightly for these exercises. When you feel ready, straighten the legs completely for a more challenging movement. As with all of the other exercises in the Daily Dozen, the key is good posture, so begin by engaging the core muscles. In both of these exercises, you should have a neutral spine (see sidebar on next page).

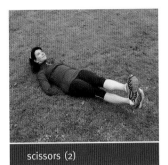
scissors (2)

STEAM ENGINE ON BACK

How to do it: Lie on your back with your hands behind your head, head slightly raised, taking care not to pull on your neck. Extend your legs fully, holding them an inch or so off the ground. Bend the left knee in toward your body as you extend your right elbow to touch the left knee. Alternate the movement, touching your right knee to your left elbow as you extend the left leg fully. **Notes:** Also known as the Bicycle, this movement is very similar to the first exercise in the Daily Dozen, the Steam Engine. It's a simple movement: bring one knee up to the opposing elbow while extending the opposite leg as far out as you can at the same time. The best way to raise the quality of this exercise is to reach the extended leg as far out as you can. This is a fantastic exercise for the abdominal muscles, the lower back, and the hamstrings.

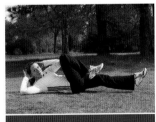
neutral spine

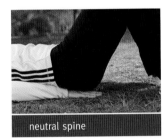
steam engine on back

PLANK

How to do it: Get into a Plank position by supporting your body weight on your elbows and lower arms and toes, with your midsection lifted and held very firm and

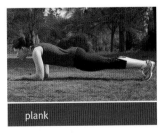
plank

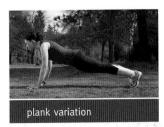
plank variation

neutral spine

Neutral spine can be best described as placing equal tension on the front and back of your body—in other words, your abdominals and lower back muscles work equally hard, and you're not favoring one side of your body or the other. To see if you're in neutral spine position, lie on the floor face up. You should be able to slide only your fingers underneath the small of your back. If the back is pressed to the ground, there's too much tension in the abdominals; if there's too much of an arch in your back, allowing room for more than your whole hand or forearm, there's probably too much tension in the back.

strong. Hold this posture for 45 seconds if you can—and challenge yourself by holding it even longer once you have the hang of it. When you're really going strong, try raising one arm or one leg—or one arm and the opposing leg at the same time—for a portion of the movement.

Variation: Try the plank with your hands on the ground, instead of your elbows.

Notes: The Plank is a very simple, smart exercise. It can be done either with the elbows on the ground, or in the Push-up position—in other words, the beginning posture of a traditional Push-up. It's often referred to in military circles as the watching TV exercise, because when you do it with your elbows on the ground, you look like a kid propped up watching television. Simply get into the position and hold it for a predetermined amount of time. Your goal for the Daily Dozen should be for 45 seconds or longer. Your body should be firm, not sagging; if the body sags, or your butt pushes up into the air, you've reached your limit.

Start doing the Daily Dozen today and you'll instantly add six hours of exercise every month. *That's* efficiency—and it will pay off in the workouts to come.

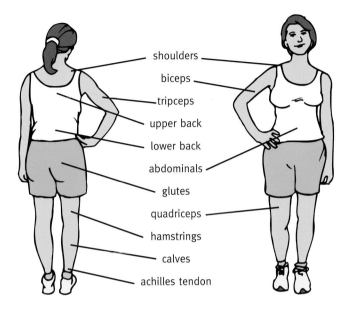

shoulders

biceps

tripceps

upper back

lower back

abdominals

glutes

quadriceps

hamstrings

calves

achilles tendon

THE HOME STRETCH

The Home Stretch is exactly what it sounds like: the last bit of your workout, the brief but essential stretching routine that will keep your muscles limber and strong. The routine starts at your toes and stretches to the top of your head and as far as your fingertips can reach.

UPPER CALF STRETCH

Starting position: Begin this stretch in the Downward Dog yoga posture: hands and feet flat on the ground, torso arched with rear up in the air, legs straight. If the Downward Dog position is uncomfortable, perform this stretch by leaning forward against a wall or another source of support, such as a tree or building, with arms straight and hands flat against the surface with legs straight and heels on the ground.

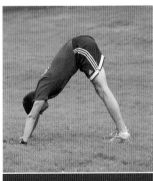

upper calf stretch (1)

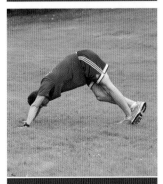

upper calf stretch (2)

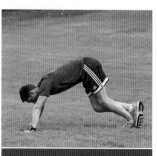

lower calves and ankles

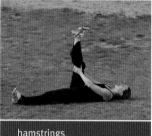

hamstrings

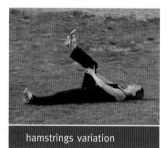

hamstrings variation

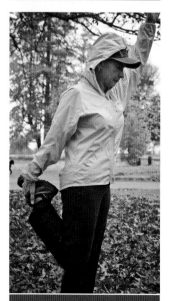

quadriceps variation

Movement: Place your left ankle above and behind the right ankle, just off the ground, so that you can feel an isolated stretch in your right calf. Keep your knee straight so as to isolate the gastrocnemius—one of two major muscles that comprise the calf. Hold this stretch for 20 seconds. Switch sides.

LOWER CALVES AND ANKLES

Starting position: Same as the Upper Calf Stretch—Downward Dog or the variation leaning against a wall.
Movement: Move your left ankle above and behind your right ankle as in the Upper Calf Stretch, with one difference: bend your right knee to isolate the soleus muscle in the lower part of your calf. Hold the stretch for 20 seconds. Switch sides.

HAMSTRINGS

Starting position: Lie on your back with your legs extended straight out in front of you. Rest your head on the ground.
Movement: Raise your right leg, with a slightly bent knee if needed. Grasp the back of your upper leg (hamstrings) with both of your hands and gently pull toward the center of your body until you feel a stretch in the hamstring. Hold for 20 seconds. Switch sides.

QUADRICEPS

Starting position: Lie flat on your stomach, chin on the ground and arms at your sides.
Movement: Raise your right ankle by bending your right knee. Grasp it behind your back with your right hand, then gently pull toward the center of your body until you feel a gentle stretch in the quadriceps muscles (the front of the thigh). Hold for 20 seconds. Switch sides.
Variation: If lying down on your stomach is uncomfortable, do this stretch standing up. Hold on to a tree or

other support with your free hand, if necessary, as you grasp your ankle and gently pull it toward your body.

HIP FLEXORS

Starting position: Sit in a kneeling position with your left leg forward. Your right knee and left foot will be on the ground, with both knees bent at 90-degree angles.

Movement: Imagine that your pelvis is a bowl of water on a table. Now, think of gently tipping the water out of the bowl from the back as you gently press the bottom part of your pelvis forward and the top part of your pelvis slightly back so that you feel a stretch in the muscles that connect the front of your hip to your right leg. That subtle tipping will activate the hip flexor in the front of your right leg. Hold for 20 seconds. Switch sides.

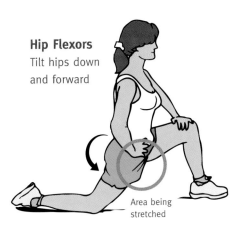

Hip Flexors
Tilt hips down and forward

Area being stretched

ILIOTIBIAL (IT) BANDS

Starting position: Stand upright near a tree, wall, or other surface for balance. Cross your right leg over your left leg.

Movement: Extend your left arm to the surface for balance. Bend your body to the left with your right arm extended overhead, as though you're doing a variation on the Side Bender from the Daily Dozen. Your goal is to feel a deep stretch in your right hip extending down to the outer part of your right leg.

Variation: Try the Pigeon Stretch if you're particularly

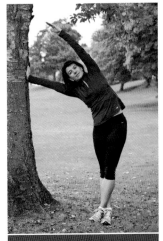

iliotibial bands

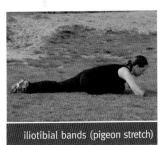

iliotibial bands (pigeon stretch)

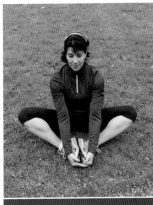

thigh adductors

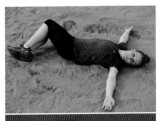

back stretch

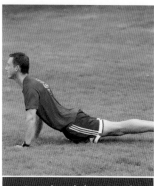
stomach and chest stretch

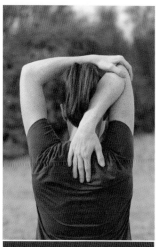
triceps stretch

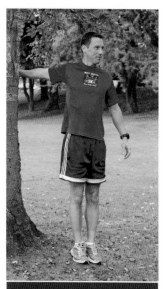
shoulder stretch

flexible. Sit on the ground and bend your left leg so that the heel is near the right hip. Extend the right leg straight behind you.

THIGH ADDUCTORS
Starting position: Sit upright with legs bent and heels placed together in front of you.
Movement: Gently press your knees toward the ground to feel a stretch in the adductors (inner thighs). Hold for 20 seconds.

BACK STRETCH
Starting position: Lie down on your back with knees bent and feet on the ground.
Movement: Gently move your knees to the left, placing them on the ground, making sure to also keep your shoulders on the ground. You should feel a stretch in your middle and lower back. Extend your arms to either side, and move your head so that you are looking to the right (away from your bent knees). Hold for 20 seconds. Switch sides.

STOMACH AND CHEST STRETCH
Starting position: Lie on your stomach, palms placed on the ground on either side of your chest, directly below your shoulders.
Movement: Look up toward the sky, gently curving your back while supporting your weight, hands on the ground. This is popularly known as the Cobra pose in yoga. Hold for 20 seconds.

TRICEPS STRETCH
Starting position: Stand upright or sit on your knees with your upper body strong and straight. Lift your left arm above your head and bend the left elbow to stretch the left triceps muscles.
Movement: Place your right hand on your left elbow to

support the stretch, gently pressing the elbow back until you feel the muscle stretching. Hold for 20 seconds. Switch sides.

SHOULDER STRETCH

Starting position: Stand near a tree or another support. Place your left hand on the support, with your left arm fully extended.
Movement: Without moving your feet, rotate your body to the right until you feel a stretch in your left shoulder and the left side of your chest. Hold for 20 seconds. Switch sides.

FINAL BREATHING

To finish the Home Stretch, take five full breaths. First, exhale and deeply Squat to the ground, arms downward. Inhale by pushing up on your heels, extending your legs, and reaching your arms to the sky. Take these breaths very slowly and deliberately—you're bringing relaxation into all areas of your body at the end of your workout, setting the tone for the next stage peacefully and with a great workout behind you.

ADDITIONAL STRETCH: CHILD'S POSE

For an additional relaxing stretch at any point during the Home Stretch, try this classic yoga posture. Sit on your heels and bend your upper body forward until your fore-head is on the ground. You can either extend your arms in front of you, or tuck them behind you next to your heels. Breathe easily and naturally as you hold this stretch.

THE WORKOUT ROUTINES

One of the four starting blocks of this program is the variety of routines you'll embark upon. Below, I describe each type of workout you'll see in your weekly workout programs.

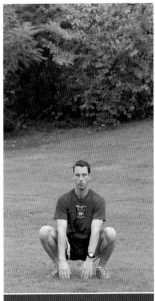
final breathing (1)

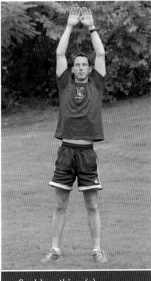
final breathing (2)

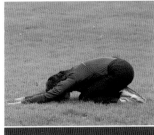
child's pose

CORNERSTONE WORKOUT

Your weekly Cornerstone Workout is the main workout of the week, lasting from 90 minutes to 2 hours. (I usually do mine on a Saturday, but you can easily adapt this to your schedule.) You'll find detailed instructions on how to do each Cornerstone Workout in the weekly workout chapters starting in the following section.

CARDIOVASCULAR ENDURANCE WORKOUT

Your Cardiovascular Endurance Workout is the longest one you'll do at moderate intensity during the week. Because different people train for different goals, you can decide how long to perform your workout on these days. A 3-hour workout is appropriate for someone training for a multiday hike or mountain climbing trip. A 45-minute fast walk is appropriate for someone just starting out. It can be any type of cardio activity that you want: running, biking, hiking, swimming, fast walking—or a combination. The key to this workout is that it is always done at a moderate pace—you should be able to carry on a conversation while performing your weekly Cardiovascular Endurance Workout.

CROSS-TRAINING WORKOUT

For the first three weeks, your Cross-Training Workout will be simple: on your regular cross-training day, you'll do the Daily Dozen with a twist, adding 2 minutes of cardio exercise (running, jumping rope, jumping jacks, fast walking, or a run/walk) between each exercise. That will add 22 minutes of cardio to your Daily Dozen—a perfect Cross-Training Workout—that mixes body weight exercises for strength-building with cardiovascular training. From Week 4 onward, cross-training will consist of any activity that supports your overall training program, meaning a combination of cardio and strength training. It could be a yoga class, kickboxing, soccer, cycling, or swimming—anything that supports your overall goals. The best cross-training exercise is the one you're actually going to do, so make it something you look forward to doing.

Another way to create a shorter Cross-Training Workout would be to take any of the Cornerstone Workouts from this book and simply cut it in half, so that you're working out for an hour or so. Personalizing your approach to your own twelve-week program makes it what you want—and that will increase your enthusiasm for getting outside and actually doing it.

TEMPO WORKOUT

During the second and third phases of your twelve-week program, you'll have the opportunity to try Tempo Workouts. To create an effective Tempo Workout, start with the Daily Dozen, then do a cardiovascular workout that incorporates a period of harder effort than the Cardiovascular Endurance Workout, but not as hard as an all-out sprint. Start by running, biking, walking fast, or swimming for 10 minutes at a moderate pace to get your body fully warmed up.

Now, move to your **tempo pace**: perform your cardio activity harder than in your warmup, but easier than an all-out effort. On a scale of perceived exertion, where 1 means you're standing still and 10 means you're running an all-out sprint, shoot for a 6 or 7 to start for your tempo pace (more advanced athletes will eventually want to get to an 8 or 8 1/2). At tempo pace, it would be hard to talk to a workout partner. Experiment, and soon you'll be able to tell what a good tempo pace feels like for you.

Beginners will start with 10 minutes of tempo work, intermediate athletes will do 20 minutes, and more advanced athletes will do 30 minutes.

Finally, cool down with 10 minutes of light cardio activity, such as a jog or walk, and your Home Stretch.

See the sidebar "Endurance Cross Training: Inspiration," in Week 2, for more information on how to gauge the intensity of your workouts and to find the right tempo pace for you.

CIRCUIT TRAINING

Circuit training is one of the most powerful forms of training available. A circuit is simply a group of exercises performed one right after another with no rest, strengthening your entire body as you go. I love nothing more than a great Circuit Training workout just because of its variety, effectiveness, and ability to train all of my different muscle groups in one session. In the pages that follow, you will learn about many different ways to incorporate circuit training into your workouts.

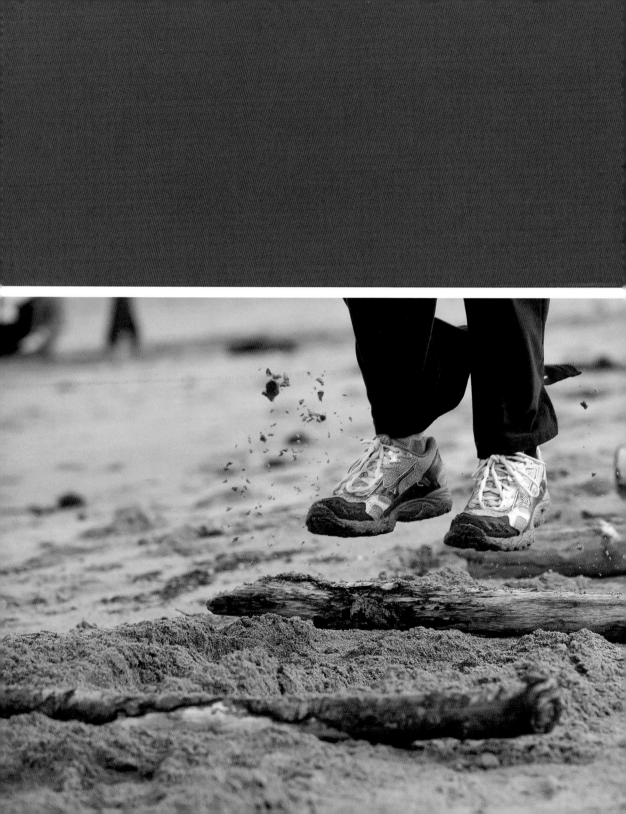

go!

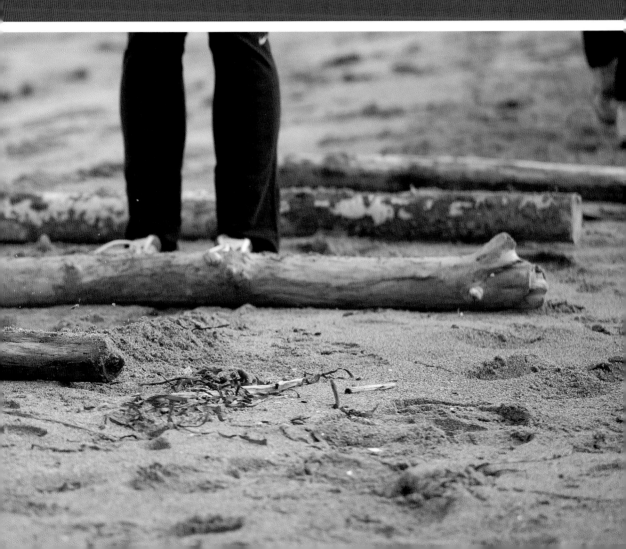

twelve weeks of
outdoor workouts

For the next twelve weeks, you'll embark upon a fitness program that might just change the way your body looks and feels. Even more important, you'll start a journey that could change the way you think about fitness and health. Sometimes you'll complete everything that is prescribed for a given day; sometimes you won't. Everyone gets tired, and we all need a break at times. We've said it before: the two most important words in fitness are *moderation* and *consistency*. The key is to keep moving, adapt the program to your own energy level, and remember that all movement counts. If you can't do ten repetitions of an exercise, do five. If you can't run, walk. If you need to stop and sit, do so. Practicing self-care is important and moderation and consistency will lead to long-term success.

START SMART: A PRECONDITIONING PROGRAM

If you haven't been active for a while, the first few weeks of this program may seem strenuous. In that case, you may wish to try a preconditioning phase before beginning the first twelve-week program. If you've had prior injuries, you might also want to work with an athletic trainer or a physical therapist who can instruct you on proper exercise technique before delving into this program.

A preconditioning program would include performing some general cardiovascular activity for 30 minutes, two to three times a week. Listen to your body. If you feel out of shape, a 10- to 15-minute walk is a good place to start; build in increments from there. On the other days of the week, perform gentle calisthenics to get your body accustomed to strength exercises.

Try the Daily Dozen, but if the exercises feel too strenuous, perform gentle movements such as leg swings, arm swings, push-ups off a wall, and squats. You could also look into pool-based aerobics classes or swimming at a local community center.

Try the following preconditioning workout for one month, and then see how you feel before trying out the full program. Include the Home Stretch five days out of seven each week (morning or evening; whatever works for your schedule) in addition to the gentle exercises suggested below:

PHASE	PRECONDITIONING
DAY 1	Daily Dozen
DAY 2	Daily Dozen; 30-minute walk
DAY 3	Rest
DAY 4	Daily Dozen; 30-minute walk, easy swim, or easy bike
DAY 5	Daily Dozen
DAY 6	Rest
DAY 7	Daily Dozen; 30–40 minute walk

tracking fitness milestones

A workout log will do wonders for your motivation and enthusiasm, as long as you make it informative and fun—and as long as you track your efforts consistently. When you jot down a timed run here or a set of Push-ups there, you might not imagine that over time, your log will provide a clear picture of your progress. It's a great source of inspiration as well. Your log can include information on anything you'd like to track: nutrition, moods, sleep patterns, and so on. As you collect information over the weeks about how you're feeling and performing in your workouts, it will inspire you to keep going.

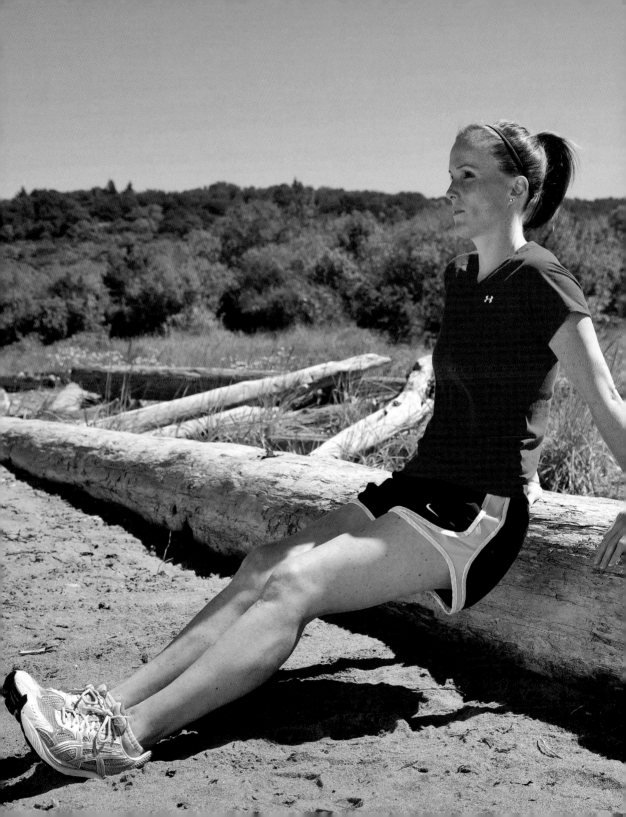

week 1 opening day

Our first training week: a little lighter, a little shorter, just enough to whet your appetite for what's to come.

WEEK 1: FIRST NOTES

The first week of your outdoor fitness program is a big deal. You might think of it as the first day of the rest of your life as an athlete—or you might struggle with the idea of calling yourself an athlete at all. Wherever you are, embrace it and go forward. This process can only fail in two circumstances: if you quit, or if you hurt yourself. Taking things at a slower pace until you're used to the increased exertion of the workouts will help you to stay healthy.

As you move through your first workout week, focus on the following:
- **Good posture:** Stand tall and strong, lengthening your body from your center. This provides stability and insurance against mishap and injury.
- **Natural movement:** Move through your fullest range of motion.
- **Movement in various directions:** Pay attention as you move forward, backward, and sideways in each of these workouts, increasing your awareness of your body's natural flow and movement.

WEEK 1: WORKOUT CHART

WEEK 1	TOTAL MINUTES	EXERCISE AND INTENSITY	MINUTES PER ROUTINE
Day 1	35–75	**Daily Dozen**	12
		Cardiovascular Endurance Moderate intensity (running, biking, hiking, swimming, fast walking, or a combination)	20–60
Day 2	12	**Daily Dozen/Rest**	12
Day 3	45–75	**Daily Dozen** *Optional walk* *or Optional yoga (any style)*	12 *30–60* *30–60*
Day 4	50	**Daily Dozen**	12
		Cross Train: Daily Dozen plus 2 minutes of cardio exercise between each routine (running, jumping rope, jumping jacks, fast walking, run/walk, or similar)	35
		Home Stretch	10
Day 5	45–75	**Daily Dozen** *Optional walk* *or Optional yoga (any style)*	12 *30–60* *30–60*
Day 6	12	**Daily Dozen/Rest**	12
Day 7	90	**Cornerstone Workout: Opening Day**	90

opening day: inspiration

If I can ask one thing of you in this first Cornerstone Workout, it's this: *Enjoy yourself.* Today is the first day of the rest of your fitness life. Putting pressure on yourself to achieve a certain mark or performance is something you may choose to do after many weeks or months of solid training, but by no means is it something to try in your first workout. Train to the best of your ability, remember the Challenge by Choice concept, and notice everything around you in the natural world.

This workout is as much about creating a relationship with your surroundings as it is about the actual physical requirements of the day. As you go through the first twelve-week cycle, you may find that you're so enamored of your outdoor surroundings that you're distracted enough to work harder than you ever imagined. (Think of how slowly time moves when you're on a treadmill in the gym—you might find that you have just the opposite experience outdoors.)

WEEK 1: DAY BY DAY

DAY 1

Now is the time to make the **Daily Dozen** as natural an extension of your morning routine as brushing your teeth or pouring that first cup of coffee. Refer to the instructions and photographs on pages 67–74 to make sure that you establish and practice the correct form for these exercises.

Select a **cardiovascular endurance activity** that you can enjoy outside, ideally with friends, for 20 to 60 minutes—perhaps a group bike ride or run, a day hike, or a spirited walk through the park. Do this activity at moderate intensity; you should be able to carry on a conversation comfortably at all times. Remember to focus on moderation and consistency—be sure not to push too far, too fast.

DAY 2

Start your day with the **Daily Dozen.** From that point forward, this is your **restoration and relaxation** day; take the time for a relaxing walk, stretch, or anything that helps you to take care of yourself.

DAY 3

In the morning, slip out of bed and right into the **Daily Dozen**. Set aside time during the day for some additional **light exercise:** a walk in your favorite park, to the grocery store, or through the neighborhood after dinner. If the weather is uncooperative or you've had a crazy day, try a light stretching exercise routine indoors, such as yoga or Pilates, a swim at the local pool, or a half hour on a cardio machine at the local gym if that's something that appeals to you.

DAY 4

Schedule an hour today for an outdoor Cross-Training Workout. Remember that your cross-training sessions are meant to combine different types of movement into a single workout. This helps your body to develop strength, flexibility, and balance, while keeping it from getting used to (or bored with) any one type of routine.

Start with the **Daily Dozen.** Then, move into the **Cross-Training Workout,** which is based on the Daily Dozen. For each Daily Dozen exercise, perform the movement for 45 seconds, rest for 15 seconds, and then spend 2 minutes doing a cardiovascular activity of your choice: running, jumping rope, jumping jacks, fast walking, cycling, or a run/walk. Repeat with the next Daily Dozen exercise until you have completed the entire routine. Finish with your **Home Stretch.**

the timed run

The timed run will help you to discover just how much faster and fitter you're getting as the weeks progress. Your challenge for this Cornerstone Workout is to find an area for a timed run, which will be a staple of your weekly workout program; you'll do it several times during the next twelve weeks to gauge your fitness progress.

This area can be a running or hiking trail, a street or sidewalk in your neighborhood, a track, a point-to-point course on a beach—anything you like. The important thing is that it be a distance you can run or run/walk in 5 to 10 minutes, and that it be a place you can return to in later weeks. It's not important to measure the exact distance; just choose a path that you can use again to time yourself in future weeks to gauge your fitness.

DAY 5

Repeat the routine from Day 3: the **Daily Dozen** and then some **light exercise** such as a brisk walk, easy swim or bike ride, yoga, or something similar.

DAY 6

Start your day with the **Daily Dozen**. For the rest of the day, give your body a well-deserved day of **restoration and relaxation**.

DAY 7

Today is your big day—your first **Cornerstone Workout**. Set aside about 1 hour and 30 minutes for an invigorating outdoor experience. Details below.

OPENING DAY: THE CORNERSTONE WORKOUT

The purpose of the Opening Day Cornerstone Workout is to introduce and practice fundamental movements that will create results, establish good habits, help prevent injury, and ensure that you maximize your workout to exercise in the most efficient way.

As you go through today's Cornerstone Workout, think of a dancer in full flight, a sprinter's arms pumping and legs reaching, or the branches of a tree swaying side to side in a storm. Consider how you can move to the fullest expression of yourself as you explore the ranges of motion introduced to you in this workout. You'll build on this knowledge as the weeks progress.

Today, focus on keeping a uniform pace. The benefit of this workout is that it taxes the cardiovascular system significantly, but not to a maximum level of exertion or to the point of excessive fatigue. You'll work hard, but not too hard, and you'll gain significant physical benefits while allowing your body to gradually get used to a new level of challenge. In future weeks, you will be outdoors for around 2 hours for the Cornerstone Workout, but today's workout is shorter—right around 90 minutes before your cooldown and Home Stretch.

Read through the entire Cornerstone Workout first to learn what activities you'll do and the ideal terrain for each set. Gather any needed gear and scout out locations so you know exactly where you're going. Don't worry if your surroundings don't provide the ideal terrain for every exercise—just use what's available, to the best of your ability.

GEAR LIST:

- Sports watch for checking the time devoted to each routine, and for clocking the timed run.
- Notepad, to record the results of your timed run (and for other notes).
- Water and energy bars, gels or another carbohydrate-rich food (you'll likely get hungry before the end of this workout).
- Your first-aid kit, cell phone, and if necessary, sunscreen and sunglasses.

IDEAL TERRAIN:

- A grassy area or similar surface (an asphalt playground, hard-packed sand in a playground, or a sandy beach at low tide) where you can perform the Daily Dozen and related exercises, standing upright and on the ground.
- A park bench, staircase, or other raised area for performing Triceps Dips (if none is available, modify the movement by performing it on the ground).
- A place where you can do a **point-to-point timed run or fast walk** of about 5 to 10 minutes, depending on your starting fitness level. (See the sidebar "The Timed Run" for more information.)

Note: For all location choices, take stock of the weather conditions in that terrain. If it's hot, find shade or a breeze; if it's cold, find sun or some sort of shelter from the wind.

THE EXERCISES:

- For the Daily Dozen exercises, turn to page 67.
- For the Home Stretch exercises, turn to page 75.
- For all other exercises, turn to Appendix A, "Compendium of Exercises," page 223.

THE CORNERSTONE WORKOUT: MINUTE BY MINUTE

00:00 to 00:15
Walk or run lightly for 5 minutes to the area you've chosen as your Daily Dozen location. Relax for a minute or two and then perform your **Daily Dozen,** doing 10 repetitions per exercise instead of 1 minute per exercise.

🕐 **00:15 to 00:25**
Run or walk for another 10 minutes. If you'd like to run the whole way but aren't used to running for a full 10 minutes, break it into two 5-minute segments, with a couple of minutes of rest in between. You can make your destination an asphalt playground or hard packed sand (as on a beach at low tide), or you could simply run for 5 minutes away from your Daily Dozen location and then run back. (Ideally make your stopping point a place with a bench, log, or a staircase for performing Triceps Dips. If none is available, you can perform the dips on the ground.)

🕐 **00:25 to 00:35**
Perform the following **sequence of 10 exercises.** These are some of the basic movements that will become a key part of your overall fitness routine.

Start with the following lower-body exercises.
- Squats—10 reps
- Lunges (static or walking forward, alternating legs)—10 reps
- Side Lunges—10 reps
- Mountain Climbers—10 reps
- Squats—10 reps

Next, perform the following warmup sequence for arms.
- Arm Circles—10 reps
- Arm Chops—10 reps
- Arm Extenders—10 reps

Next, move on to strength exercises for the upper body.
- Push-ups—1 set of 12 reps performed as follows: 2 reps, 10 seconds rest, 4 reps, 10 seconds rest, 6 reps.
  Note: For the rest between the Push-ups sets, you can practice Child's Pose, Downward Dog, or simply rest in the Push-up start position with your knees on the ground—a front-leaning rest position.
- Triceps Dips (on a bench or raised area, or on the ground)—10 reps.

🕐 **00:35 to 00:45**
Get ready for your timed run. **Jog or walk lightly** for 10 minutes. End at the area you've designated for the timed run.

00:45 to 00:50
Take a moment to do a few **warmup exercises** before you start the run.
Perform each of the following movements for about 10 seconds and repeat
the entire circuit twice, for a total of 2 to 3 minutes of warming up. This will
prepare you for the run and for the added stress of a harder effort.

- Butt Kicks
- Side-to-Side Strides
- High Knees
- Backwards Running
- Skipping
- Skipping with High Knees
- Gazelles

Return to the starting point and rest completely for 2 minutes.

00:50 to 01:00
Perform your timed run (or run/walk) on your designated course. Set your
sports watch and then time yourself as you run or walk the distance you
have marked. Try to bring your intensity level to a moderately high level. Run
or walk at a pace that makes it difficult to hold a conversation comfortably,
but don't make an all-out effort. Be aggressive yet conservative and you'll
post a time for this run that you can use to compare your fitness level over
time. Jot it down in your notebook.

01:00 to 01:15
Take a short **rest** after the timed run, with water and an energy snack or gel
if you're hungry. **Cool down** by doing an easy walk/run for 3 to 5 minutes, to
keep your muscles moving as you ramp down. Your destination should be
a soft surface where you can comfortably perform exercises on the ground.
When you feel ready to move on, perform the following set of **core exercises**
for 10 repetitions each, with 15 seconds of rest after each exercise:

- Crocodiles—10 reps
- Scissors—10 reps
- Steam Engines on Back—10 reps
- Russian Twists—10 reps
- Push-outs—10 reps

Take 1 minute of rest, and then repeat the sequence in its entirety. Finish with a set of 10 Burpees—one of our favorite exercises for building core strength, endurance, and quickness.

1:15 to 1:30
The final "push" for the Opening Day Cornerstone Workout is a set of 1-minute runs interspersed with 10 exercises. If you're not already at the location where you began today's workout, you can run toward that location for each of the 10 minutes you'll run during this sequence.

- Push-ups—10 reps
- Run 1 minute
- Arm Extenders—10 reps
- Run 1 minute
- Mountain Climbers—10 reps
- Run 1 minute
- Squats—10 reps
- Run 1 minute
- Burpees—10 reps
- Run 1 minute
- Plank—30 seconds
- Run 1 minute
- Squats—10 reps
- Run 1 minute
- Lunges—10 reps
- Run 1 minute
- Calf Raises—10 reps
- Run 1 minute
- Russian Twists—10 reps
- Run 1 minute

01:30 to 01:40
Perform the **Home Stretch**. Congratulations—you've made it through Opening Day.

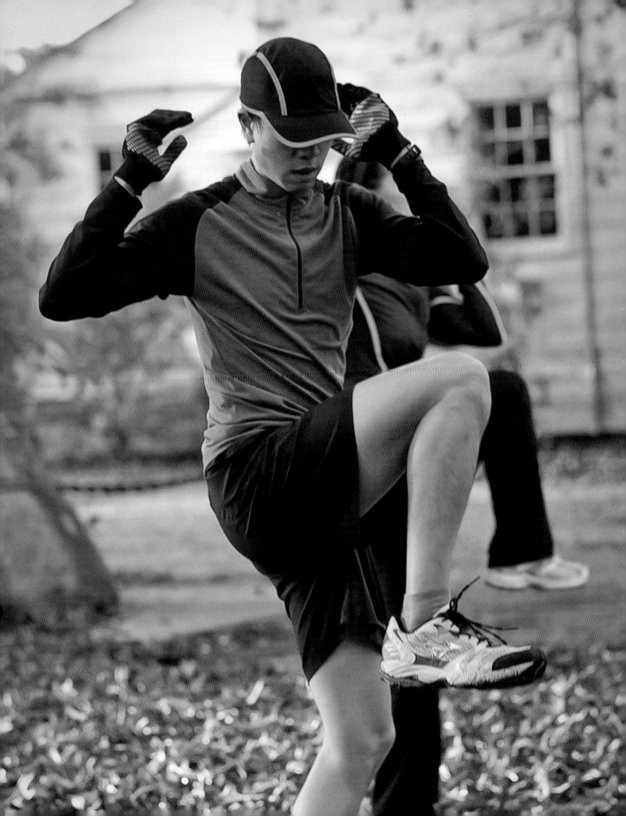

week 2 endurance cross-training

By now, you're building more endurance. This week, you'll do the same workout on days 1 through 6 as you did last week, and then in your Cornerstone Workout, you'll pair longer, slower aerobic intervals with strength-building sessions for a complete overall workout.

WEEK 2: FIRST NOTES

The daily routine for Week 2 is identical to Week 1 except for the Cornerstone Workout, which introduces Endurance Cross-Training (EXT for short). EXT is all about keeping your body moving for an extended period of time, while performing challenging cross-training activities to systematically strengthen each muscle group and system. EXT creates an understanding of different levels of exercise intensity and the energy systems that are recruited by the body to work at different levels of effort. Focus this week on core movements such as the Squat and Push-up, and work to increase your concentration on movement and proper form.

WEEK 2: WORKOUT CHART

WEEK 2	TOTAL MINUTES	EXERCISE AND INTENSITY	MINUTES PER ROUTINE
Day 1	35–75	**Daily Dozen**	12
		Cardiovascular Endurance Moderate intensity (running, biking, hiking, swimming, fast walking, or a combination)	20–60
Day 2	12	**Daily Dozen/Rest**	12
Day 3	45–75	**Daily Dozen** *Optional walk* *or Optional yoga (any style)*	12 *30–60* *30–60*
Day 4	50	**Daily Dozen**	12
		Cross Train: Daily Dozen plus 2 minutes of cardio exercise between each routine (running, jumping rope, jumping jacks, fast walking, run/walk, or similar)	35
		Home Stretch	10
Day 5	45–75	**Daily Dozen** *Optional walk* *or Optional yoga (any style)*	12 *30–60* *30–60*
Day 6	12	**Daily Dozen/Rest**	12
Day 7	120	**Cornerstone Workout: Endurance Cross-Training**	120

WEEK 2: DAY BY DAY

DAY 1
Start with the **Daily Dozen**. Continue your workout with a moderate **cardiovascular endurance** activity: running, biking, swimming, or another activity for 20 to 60 minutes, depending on your fitness and energy level today.

DAY 2
Start your day with the **Daily Dozen.** Make the rest of the day a **restoration and relaxation** day with a massage, walk, light stretching routine, or anything else that helps you to take care of yourself.

DAY 3
Begin with your **Daily Dozen.** If your body feels up for it, take 30 to 60 minutes for **a brisk walk outside or do some yoga exercises.** Any yoga style will do; the goal here is to simply increase the variety in your routine. Yoga provides a great way to stretch your body and relax your mind; I recommend working a class into your weekly schedule if time and money permits, or simply get a DVD from your local library and follow along.

DAY 4
Today is your Daily Dozen/Cross-Training Workout day. Start with the **Daily Dozen.** Next, do the **Cross-Training Workout** from Week 1: perform the exercises in the Daily Dozen, incorporating 2 minutes of cardio activity such as running, jumping rope, jumping jacks, fast walking, or a run/walk between each Daily Dozen exercise. This should feel a bit like a mini version of the Cornerstone Workout—quicker and less intense, but still a challenge.

DAY 5
Repeat the routine from Day 3: the **Daily Dozen**, and then some **light exercise** such as a walk, yoga, or something similar.

DAY 6
Start your day with the **Daily Dozen.** For the rest of the day, give your body a well-deserved day of **restoration and relaxation.**

endurance cross-training: inspiration

What does a car's revolution counter have to do with your body? On that counter, there's a red line that signifies the difference between sustainable and unsustainable speeds. Like a car, if the body isn't warmed up properly, going over the red line will be detrimental to long-term performance. The human body has a red line: the *anaerobic threshold*. It's the level of effort where lactate, a by-product of exercise, accumulates in your blood at a concentration higher than what can be simultaneously expended. At that level of exertion, you'll get tired very, very quickly.

Anaerobic threshold is the dividing line between two levels of intensity. The first is the level where you are supplying sufficient oxygen to your body to maintain a moderate effort. This is aerobic exercise, from the Greek *aer* ("in the presence of oxygen"). The second level is anaerobic, "without the presence of oxygen." Here, your body requires more oxygen to work the muscles and brain than your heart and lungs can supply. When you practice endurance activities such as running or cycling, the majority of the effort will be within aerobic limits. However, in interval training, for brief periods of time you will reach your anaerobic threshold. (If you feel out of breath, you've likely reached that threshold.)

On a **scale of perceived exertion**, where 1 means you're standing still and 10 means you're running an all-out sprint, you're likely to reach your anaerobic threshold somewhere between 7 and 9.

When you train correctly, your anaerobic threshold will increase, meaning you can do more work before reaching that threshold. Simply put, you will become a better athlete. After a few weeks on this program you will likely have a higher anaerobic threshold, as well as other benefits. You will be able to move faster and further in your comfort zone, and with the overall higher fitness level, you can dip into the anaerobic zone with more frequency and vigor.

This week's Cornerstone Workout occurs well below the red line, with one exception—your timed run. Definitely run hard if you feel ready for it in your timed run, but for the rest of the workout, consider going slower than what you might think the "right" pace is. That will allow you to go much longer as you work on your endurance. According to exercise physiologists and professional coaches, far more athletes overtrain than undertrain. It's very important to know that you should not leave each workout feeling exhausted, but that your goal should be to leave the workout feeling invigorated, energized, happy, and strong.

DAY 7

Today is your **Endurance Cross-Training Cornerstone Workout.** Details follow.

ENDURANCE CROSS-TRAINING: THE CORNERSTONE WORKOUT

As you begin this week's Cornerstone Workout, consider *movement awareness*. Think in terms of your body's full range of motion: you can bend forward and back from your waist, or side to side, and you can twist. As you train, think about each exercise and the type of movement you're using to gradually increase awareness of your body. You will grow more aware of how your body is feeling, and what the appropriate workload is for you.

Another goal of this workout is to *celebrate* your body the way a dancer celebrates the expression of movement.

GEAR LIST:

- Your usual kit: a sports watch, water, energy snack, small notebook and pen, first-aid kit, cell phone, and sun protection if necessary.
- Six cones or rocks to mark stations for the In-Line Circuit workout. (Optional: find rocks when you get to your In-Line Circuit location, or carry cones in a small backpack.)

IDEAL TERRAIN:

- A sand pit or a grassy field for your In-Line Circuit.
- Your timed run path.
- Stairs or a hill, if available.

THE EXERCISES:

- For the Daily Dozen exercises, turn to page 67.
- For the Home Stretch exercises, turn to page 75.
- For all other exercises, turn to Appendix A, "Compendium of Exercises," page 223.

ENDURANCE CROSS-TRAINING: MINUTE BY MINUTE

🕐 **00:00 to 00:20**
Begin with a **warmup run or run/walk** for 5 minutes. Run among trees if possible, touching as many as you can while moving your body. Next, do your **Daily Dozen.**

🕐 **00:20 to 00:25**
Run or run/walk to either a sand pit, if one is available, or a grassy field.

🕐 **00:25 to 00:35**
Perform the following **In-Line Circuit**. You'll see the circuit in several places over the next few workouts: it's a mixture of agility exercises using cones, rocks, or other objects to set up the course; calisthenics; and running. We call it an "in-line" circuit because you perform the exercises one right after the other, with no rest in between exercises. If a sand pit or a soccer field is not available, you can set this circuit up in a backyard or even a playground. Use your imagination.

The In-Line Circuit should feel like a game. enjoy the sense of constant movement as you go from one exercise station to the next. Place six cones or rocks a short distance apart from one another (about 100 feet) in any pattern you wish (oval, square, straight line) to designate the stations for each exercise in the circuit. Make a starting point, get out a watch, set your timer for 10 minutes, and go! Your task is to complete the circuit as many times as you can, at moderate intensity, within the 10-minute period. (If you don't have cones or rocks available to mark the locations for each exercise, simply run about 100 feet between exercises.)

Perform 10 repetitions each of the following exercises, repeating as many circuits as you can, for 10 minutes straight:

▌ Burpees
▌ Push-ups
▌ Squats
▌ Mountain Climbers
▌ Triceps Dips
▌ Jumping Jacks

🕐 **00:35 to 00:45**
Run or run/walk for 10 minutes to a grassy area for a Core Superset—50 consecutive repetitions of strength exercises for your core muscles.

🕐 **00:45 to 00:55**
Core Superset. Perform 10 repetitions of each exercise:
- Push-ups
- Russian Twists
- Ranger Crawls
- Steam Engines
- Push-outs

After this circuit, take 5 full minutes of rest before moving on to your timed run.

🕐 **01:00 to 01:10**
Timed Run. Rest for 4 to 5 minutes after completing the timed run.

🕐 **01:15 to 01:25**
In-Line Circuit. Repeat the same circuit of exercises that you did earlier in the workout for 10 minutes. Try to do the second circuit a little harder than the first.

🕐 **01:25 to 01:35**
Repeat your **timed run**. It's challenging to do this twice in one workout, so remember the Challenge by Choice concept—go as fast or as moderately as your body wants to go.

🕐 **01:35 to 01:40**
Run or run/walk to a set of stairs. If a set of stairs is not available, a hill will work.

🕐 **01:40 to 01:50**
Run or run/walk the stairs or hill (making sure to always walk, not run, down the stairs or downhill). Do this at your own pace for 10 minutes.

🕐 **01:50 to 02:00**
Home Stretch. Enjoy the rest of your day, and congratulations on completing your first EXT workout.

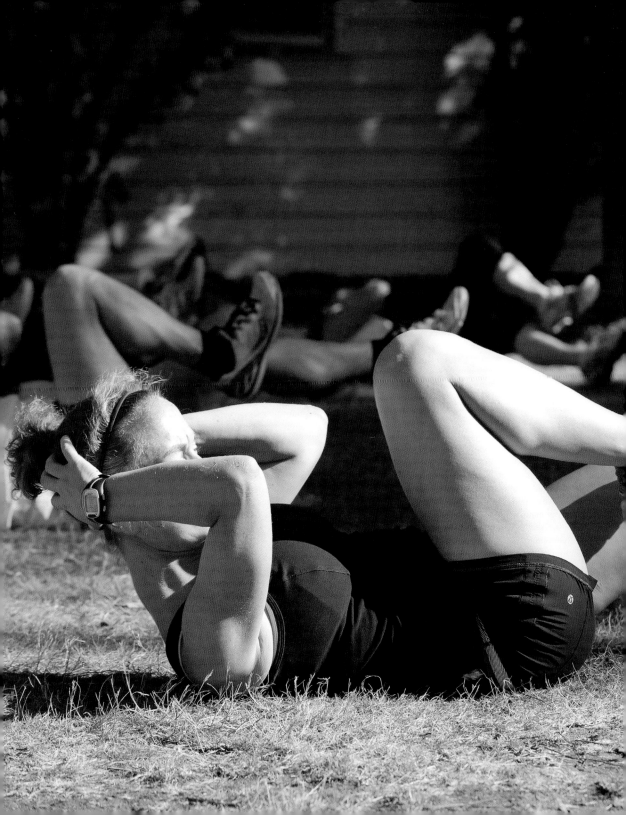

week 3 super circuits

Building on the circuits you've done for the first two weeks of the program, this week you'll dedicate an entire Cornerstone Workout to them. You'll begin the week with your basic conditioning routine, and then move to Super Circuits, our all-circuits workout, for a great challenge with excellent variety.

WEEK 3: FIRST NOTES

There are many different approaches to a Circuit Training workout, but all of the methods have something in common: performing single sets of multiple exercises in a circuit with a short amount of rest (if any) in between. You've done it for two weeks already (the Daily Dozen in itself is technically a circuit workout). This week, you'll expand on circuits even more, working on your basic conditioning during the week and then tackling two different types of circuits in your Cornerstone Workout that you can do virtually anywhere.

Circuit training is really a very basic way to exercise. Just choose your exercises, stay in motion, and you'll reap the benefits. It's something every Olympic athlete does as part of his or her training—and after this week, it will be a part of your exercise repertoire as well.

WEEK 3: WORKOUT CHART

WEEK 3	TOTAL MINUTES	EXERCISE AND INTENSITY	MINUTES PER ROUTINE
Day 1	35–75	**Daily Dozen**	12
		Cardiovascular Endurance Moderate intensity (running, biking, hiking, swimming, fast walking, or a combination)	20–60
Day 2	12	**Daily Dozen/Rest**	12
Day 3	45–75	**Daily Dozen** *Optional walk* *or Optional yoga (any style)*	12 *30–60* *30–60*
Day 4	50	**Daily Dozen**	12
		Cross Train: Daily Dozen plus 2 minutes of cardio exercise between each routine (running, jumping rope, jumping jacks, fast walking, run/walk, or similar)	35
Day 5	45–75	**Daily Dozen** *Optional walk* *or Optional yoga (any style)*	12 *30–60* *30–60*
Day 6	12	**Daily Dozen/Rest**	12
Day 7	120	**Cornerstone Workout:** **Super Circuits**	120

WEEK 3: DAY BY DAY

DAY 1
Start your day with the **Daily Dozen.** Continue your workout with a moderate **cardiovascular endurance** activity: running, biking, swimming, or another activity for 20 to 60 minutes, depending on your fitness and energy level today.

DAY 2
Start your day with the **Daily Dozen.** You've earned a rest; make sure to take time for **restoration and relaxation** for the remainder of the day.

DAY 3
Begin with your **Daily Dozen.** If your body feels up for it, take 30 to 60 minutes for a brisk walk outside, some yoga, or any other form of gentle movement.

DAY 4
Perform your **Daily Dozen with a cross-training twist**. Incorporate 2 minutes of cardio activity such as running, jumping rope, jumping jacks, fast walking, or a run/walk between each Daily Dozen exercise. As usual, expect this workout to tire you out; you should reach an intensity level of around 60 to 70 percent for much of the workout.

DAY 5
Repeat the routine from Day 3: the **Daily Dozen** and then some **light exercise** such as a walk, yoga, or something similar.

DAY 6
Start your day with the **Daily Dozen.** For the rest of the day, give your body some well-deserved **restoration and relaxation**.

DAY 7
It's time for the **Super Circuits Cornerstone Workout.**

super circuits: inspiration

Circuit training has been used in athletics as a coaching method for well over a century. In fact, in the mid-twentieth cen-tury it was predominant, being one of the most popular forms of athletic training. Since then, many fitness trends have come and gone—aerobics, step classes, Jazzercise, and the like—and now we see a resurgence of circuit training in many fitness clubs around the country. With circuit training, you work really hard for a short amount of time at an intensity that you would not be able to sustain for very long. Just at the point where you start to get tired, you rest—but that rest is just long enough to enable you to make another effort. A well-designed circuit training program provides a higher return on your exercise investment in terms of time and energy than virtually any other type of training, and allows you to add variety and intensity to your workouts.

SUPER CIRCUITS: THE CORNERSTONE WORKOUT

The purpose of the Super Circuits is to solidify the concept and practice of circuit training.

GEAR LIST:

- Your usual kit: a sports watch, water, energy snack, small notebook and pen, first-aid kit, cell phone, and sun protection if necessary.
- 20-yard rope, to measure out the shuttle run distance.
- Jump rope (optional).
- Eight cones, rocks, or other objects to mark circuit stations.

IDEAL TERRAIN:

- For the circuits, flat ground (grass, asphalt, sand, a playground, or even an indoor basketball court or other gym floor) is ideal. Note that the area you choose for the circuits doesn't need to be very large, because we won't venture far for this circuit.

THE EXERCISES:

- For the Daily Dozen exercises, turn to page 67.
- For the Home Stretch exercises, turn to page 75.
- For all other exercises, turn to Appendix A, "Compendium of Exercises," page 223.

SUPER CIRCUITS: MINUTE BY MINUTE

00:00 to 00:20
Our usual **warmup.** Run or run/walk for 5 to 10 minutes, and then perform your **Daily Dozen.**

00:20 to 00:55
Run for 10 minutes to your first circuit location. (If this is the same as your warmup location, just run for 5 minutes away from that spot, and then run back—use whatever terrain you have available.)

What follows is the **Basic Circuit**—a simple circuit workout that will become a part of your midweek workouts starting in Week 4. This circuit is made up of 8 exercises. Set up your circuit course using 8 cones or rocks, each spaced about 50 feet apart. Each cone represents a different exercise from the list below. At the first cone, perform the first exercise (Push-ups) for 40 seconds. Rest for 20 seconds, then walk or run to the next cone and perform the next exercise (Steam Engines on Back) for 40 seconds, followed by another 20 seconds of rest. Continue around the circuit course. Do **3 circuits** of these 8 exercises:

- Push-ups
- Steam Engines on Back
- Squats
- Ranger Crawls
- Jump Rope or Jumping Jacks
- Burpees
- Russian Twists
- Shuttle Run (see sidebar, page 116)

00:55 to 01:10
Take a **water break** before heading to the location for your second circuit.

You can either **run or run/walk for 5 to 10 minutes** to get to another grassy field or similar terrain, or simply run/walk in an out-and-back course to return to the original terrain for your first circuit—it will work just as well for your second circuit.

🕐 **01:10 to 01:30**

Our second circuit today is an **In-Line Circuit**. Remember that you'll perform these exercises in a constant motion (in other words, "in-line"), instead of 40 seconds on and 20 seconds off. You'll keep moving for 20 minutes straight, doing 10 reps of each exercise until the 20 minutes has elapsed. This is a great time to review your commitment to Challenge by Choice: do only as much as you're comfortable doing, pushing yourself when you feel ready to do so, but holding back if you sense your body needs to take this circuit more gradually. If you feel strong, track how many circuits you complete in the 20 minutes. Or go at a slower intensity and pay close attention to correct form. Either way, you'll see that this is a fun, challenging, and exciting way to raise your energy level toward the end of your workout. The circuit exercises are listed again below for reference.

- Push-ups
- Steam Engines on Back
- Squats
- Ranger Crawls
- Jump Rope or Jumping Jacks
- Burpees
- Russian Twists
- Shuttle Run

🕐 **01:30 to 01:40**

Cool Down. Do an easy run or run/walk for 10 minutes to your Home Stretch location.

🕐 **01:40 to 01:50**

Home Stretch. And you're done. Great job—grab a snack and enjoy the rest of your day.

more thoughts on super circuits

This workout incorporates two types of circuits: classic **circuit training** (with rest periods in between each exercise) and **in-line circuits** (where you stay in constant motion). You'll see that these are two separate types of circuit workouts that you can do anywhere, anytime, to incorporate more high-intensity training into your fitness program. With circuit training, there is no limit to the creativity you can add to the workout—simply swap out other exercises, change the reps or the time per exercise, or shorten or lengthen the circuit to alter the intensity and length of the workout. In other words, circuits are extremely adaptable. Change the circuit workout in a way that feels right for your body. It's the first step in creating your own outdoor fitness workouts tailored to your personal goals.

By selecting sport-specific exercises, you can tailor the circuit workout for specific sports and fitness goals. The circuit workout for this week is a general fitness-enhancing all-body workout exercising all of the major muscle groups. However, it is not uncommon to do a circuit training workout that focuses on a specific area of the body (legs, core, etc.), or a specific set of skills for a given sport (cycling, hiking, running, skiing, etc.). See Appendix B, "Sport-Specific Circuit Training," for some suggestions on tailoring your circuit training to your own sports goals.

week 4 put it to the test

This week, we'll push the edge of your comfort zone. You'll measure your progress, become aware of your gathering strength, and set measurable milestones for tracking your fitness progress with a fitness test.

WEEK 4: FIRST NOTES

From weeks 1 to 3, you were in your **Adaptation** phase, adapting to your new training program. In Week 4, you'll enter a four-week phase of **Building**: adding strength and endurance to your foundation. From weeks 4 to 7, you'll continue to build toward a goal of **Peaking** your performance in weeks 8 to 12. The Building phase of training adds a more challenging midweek workout—a **Tempo Workout** in which you'll perform your favorite cardio activity at a higher intensity level (70 to 80 percent of your maximum effort) for an extended period of time. On the weekend, you'll get a chance to set some new benchmarks for performance as you take your first fitness test.

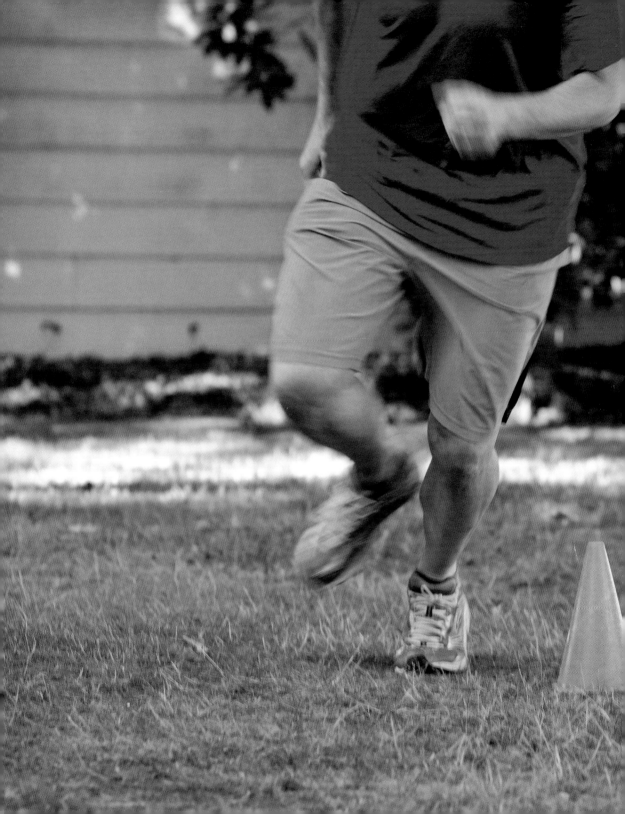

WEEK 4: WORKOUT CHART

WEEK 4	TOTAL MINUTES	EXERCISE AND INTENSITY	MINUTES PER ROUTINE
Day 1	60–135	**Daily Dozen**	12
		Cardiovascular Endurance Moderate intensity (running, biking, hiking, swimming, fast walking, or a combination)	45–120
Day 2	12	**Daily Dozen/Rest**	12
Day 3	50–55	**Circuit Training:**	
		Cardio Warmup: Run or run/walk to location for Basic Circuit	5
		Daily Dozen	12
		Basic Circuit x 3: Perform each of the following exercises for 40 seconds each, with 20 seconds of rest in between. One time through the list of exercises equals one circuit. Do 3 circuits with minimal rest in between circuits: Push-ups, Steam Engines on Back, Squats, Ranger Crawls, Jump Rope or Jumping Jacks, Burpees, Russian Twists, Shuttle Run	25
		Home Stretch	10
Day 4	55–85	**Daily Dozen**	12
		Tempo Workout: Choose a cardio activity you enjoy, such as running, fast walking, cycling, or swimming. For your Tempo Workout, do the following: **Warm Up**—10 minutes at an easy pace (around 50% of your maximum effort).	30–60

WEEK 4	TOTAL MINUTES	EXERCISE AND INTENSITY	MINUTES PER ROUTINE
		Tempo—Speed up your pace so that you are closer to 70% to 80% of your maximum effort. *Duration: Beginners—10 minutes Intermediate—20 minutes Advanced—30 minutes*	
		Cool Down—10 minutes at an easy pace	
		Or Cross Train: Daily Dozen plus 2 minutes of cardio exercise between each routine (running, jumping rope, jumping jacks, fast walking, run/walk, or similar)	
		Home Stretch	10
DAY 5	50–55	**Circuit Training:**	
		Cardio Warmup: Run or run/walk to location for Basic Circuit	5
		Daily Dozen	12
		Basic Circuit x 3: Perform each of the following exercises for 40 seconds each, with 20 seconds of rest in between. One time through the list of exercises equals one circuit. Do 3 circuits with minimal rest in between circuits: Push-ups, Steam Engines on Back, Squats, Ranger Crawls, Jump Rope or Jumping Jacks, Burpees, Russian Twists, Shuttle Run	25
		Home Stretch	10
DAY 6	12	**Daily Dozen/Rest**	12
DAY 7	120	**Cornerstone Workout: Put It to the Test**	120

the shuttle run

The Shuttle Run, which we introduced in last week's Super Circuits Cornerstone Workout, is one of four fitness tests you'll perform during this workout. It's not complicated, but it can be tricky to set up the first time around, so you may want to practice the setup beforehand just to make sure you know exactly how to perform the test during the workout. The only extra gear you'll need is a piece of rope around 20 yards long (60 feet)—and even this is optional.

To set up your Shuttle Run course, either lay the rope out end to end on a grassy field or a paved area, or simply measure out about 20 yards by taking 20 strides forward. Mark the beginning and ending points with two cones or rocks.

To perform the test, run from one cone to the other and back again as many times as you can. Count each half-lap (one time between cones) as one repetition. Run for two minutes, and record the number in your notebook.

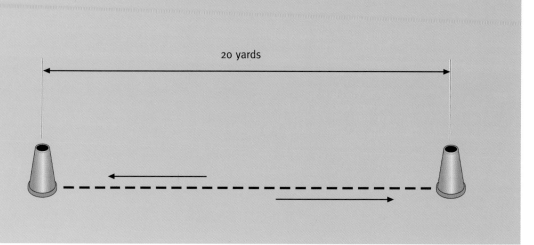

20 yards

WEEK 4: DAY BY DAY

DAY 1

Start with your **Daily Dozen**. Instead of 20 to 60 minutes, the suggested duration for your **cardiovascular endurance workout** is up to 45 to 120 minutes. Pace yourself and choose a duration that feels right to you, even if it's less than 45 minutes. Enjoy this activity at moderate intensity, as always.

DAY 2

Start with the **Daily Dozen.** From that point forward, this is your **restoration and relaxation** day; take the time for a relaxing walk, stretch, or anything that helps you to take care of yourself.

DAY 3

A new challenge: today you'll do a **circuit workout** based on the Basic Circuit from last week's Cornerstone Workout (see Day 7, "Super Circuits: The Cornerstone Workout," of Week 3). Set aside about 1 hour for this workout. **Run for 5 minutes** to a location for your circuit, perform your **Daily Dozen**, and then perform three rounds of the **Basic Circuit** (see the workout chart above for the exercise list). Finish with your **Home Stretch.**

DAY 4

Challenge by Choice: After performing your **Daily Dozen**, schedule 30 minutes to 1 hour for either a Tempo Workout or your usual outdoor Cross-Training Workout. You have choices for your **Cross-Training Workout:** do the same workout you've done so far in this program, or for variety, take one of the Cornerstone Workouts you've done so far and simply cut it in half, so that you're working out for an hour or so. If you're up for a **Tempo Workout,** choose a cardio exercise that you enjoy: running, fast walking, cycling, or swimming are ideal. Start with a warmup at moderate intensity (50 percent of your maximum effort), and then push your pace up to 70 or 80 percent of your maximum effort. Do this for 10 minutes if you're a beginner, 20 if you're an intermediate athlete, and 30 minutes if you're advanced. While you should not feel out of breath, you should feel as though this is a significant effort that requires concentration. (See the sidebar "Endurance Cross-Training: Inspiration," in Week 2, for more infomation about how to gauge the intensity of your workouts.) Finish with 10 minutes at an easy pace, and top it off with your **Home Stretch.**

put it to the test: inspiration

There are many different ways to approach an exercise program. One is to go through the motions, work out when you have time, take a class here or there, and just sweat a little bit. Lots of people do just that, wonder why they never improve their fitness or lose any significant amount of weight, and never gain much enthusiasm for exercising. Another way is practiced by those who get involved in their exercise lives, paying attention to every improvement. Most of us fall somewhere in between. Whether you've slept through 6:00 AM gym classes in the past or timed every quarter-mile you've run since grade school, **Put It to the Test** will help you discover your baseline fitness level, gaining a true sense of accomplishment as you progress knowing exactly how much you're improving. From there, it's up to you—you may wish to track multiple fitness milestones (like your time on a 1-mile run, or the number of Push-ups you can do in a single set), or the tests in this book may be enough for you. Either way, celebrate *knowing* where you really are on your fitness journey— it's meant to be a benchmark and a learning tool, not a judgment.

DAY 5

Same as Day 3: the **Basic Circuit workout. Run for 5 minutes** to a location for your circuit, perform your **Daily Dozen,** and then perform 3 rounds of the **Basic Circuit** (see the workout chart above for the exercise list). Finish with your **Home Stretch**.

DAY 6

Start your day with the **Daily Dozen**. For the rest of the day, give your body a well-deserved day of **restoration and relaxation**.

DAY 7

Time for your **Put It to the Test Cornerstone Workout.**

PUT IT TO THE TEST: THE CORNERSTONE WORKOUT

The purpose of the Put It to the Test Cornerstone Workout is to establish a baseline of fitness. Now that you've exercised in the outdoors for almost three full weeks, it's time to measure your fitness so you'll have a basis for comparison over the coming weeks. Think of this workout as a milestone workout—one in which you're measuring your fitness in very specific ways, and perhaps accomplishing more than you ever have before. In the business of rehabilitation and physical therapy, clients are recognized for completing each month of work—it's a celebration, and a big one at that, because many people don't commit to sticking with it. At adventX, we mark "birthdays" to celebrate the long-term commitments our athletes have made to bettering themselves through a lifetime of fitness. Set up a similar reward system for yourself to make your fitness journey even more fun and rewarding as the weeks progress.

GEAR LIST
▪ Your usual kit: a sports watch, water, energy snack, small notebook and pen, first-aid kit, cell phone, and sun protection if necessary.
▪ 20-yard piece of rope (optional).
▪ Two cones, rocks, or other small objects (optional).

IDEAL TERRAIN
▪ A grassy area or other flat, soft ground for your fitness tests.
▪ Your usual timed-run course.

THE EXERCISES:
▪ For the Daily Dozen exercises, turn to page 67.
▪ For the Home Stretch exercises, turn to page 75.
▪ For all other exercises, turn to Appendix A, "Compendium of Exercises," page 223.

more on fitness tests

As you cool down from this week's Cornerstone Workout, consider that the fitness test is an opportunity to bring your body to a new level of fitness, just by challenging yourself to do as much as you can. When we do this fitness test in adventX classes, it's not uncommon for athletes to do more Push-ups or have faster Shuttle Run times than ever before. Pay attention to your successes and celebrate them. See breakthroughs in these fitness tests as a recognition of your efforts over the past three weeks. Know that your commitment so far is a strong indicator of your success to come.

PUT IT TO THE TEST: MINUTE BY MINUTE

00:00 to 00:20
Run or run/walk for 5 to 10 minutes to your warmup area. Do your **Daily Dozen.**

00:20 to 01:00
Fitness Test. This will consist of your timed run and a strength test with 4 exercises designed to gauge your upper-body strength, core strength, explosiveness and endurance, and sprint speed.

Do the **timed run** first, going at a speed that feels like a solid effort. Record your time. Then, **rest** completely for 5 minutes (gentle walking or just pacing slowly back and forth).

Next, to prepare for your strength test sequence, **walk or walk/run** for an additional 3 minutes at a slightly higher intensity than on your post-timed run/walk in order to get your blood pumping and your body ready for the more intense effort to come.

For the **strength test,** find an area that has a solid, level, soft surface (grass is perfect). Avoid pavement for this strength test (with the exception of the

Shuttle Run) as you'll be performing one set of strength exercises on the ground. During this test, you will perform four exercises for 2 minutes each, with 3 minutes of rest in between each exercise. For the first three exercises, the goal will be to count the number of perfect repetitions you can complete in 2 minutes. If you do this with a partner, you can rest while counting their repetitions—along with cheering them on! For the fourth exercise, the Shuttle Run, simply time yourself. Write down your scores for each test; you'll do the whole test sequence again in Week 11 to see how far your fitness has progressed.

Perform the **strength test** as follows:

- Push-ups—2 minutes, followed by 4 minutes of rest
- Steam Engines on Back—2 minutes, followed by 4 minutes of rest
- Burpees—2 minutes, followed by 4 minutes of rest
- 20-yard Shuttle Run—Set up your shuttle run course as explained in the sidebar on page 116. Run back and forth between your cones for 2 minutes, counting the number of times you complete one repetition between the cones.

01:00 to 01:10

Cool Down. Take 5 to 10 minutes for a light run or run/walk. After a maximal effort such as these fitness tests, it's natural to feel soreness and perhaps some fatigue in the chest, lungs, legs, and arms. While "no pain, no gain" is a worn-out concept, it doesn't hurt to have a little more sensation in your body after a hard effort, knowing that you've done a great workout.

01:10 to 01:20

Home Stretch. This is a shorter program today because of the extraordinary effort you've put forth. Take special care to move through your stretches, as you've taxed your body a great deal today.

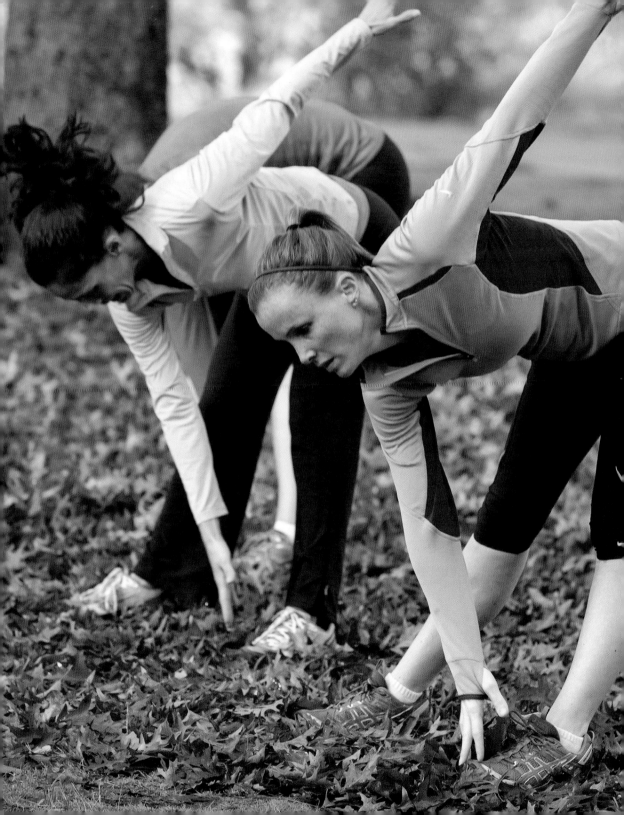

week 5 perfect balance

Can you stand on one foot? For 3 minutes straight? Neither can we—that's why we're still working on it ourselves. Join us for a week of great conditioning topped off by a Cornerstone Workout designed to give you perfect balance.

WEEK 5: FIRST NOTES

The purpose of this week is to explore balance. We'll get in a great aerobic and strength workout, coupled with specific balance-building exercises to increase your sense of your body in space and contribute to greater confidence. That could mean the difference between someday slipping and fracturing a hip—or arresting your fall and walking away with nothing more than a bruise.

WEEK 5: WORKOUT CHART

WEEK 5	TOTAL MINUTES	EXERCISE AND INTENSITY	MINUTES PER ROUTINE
Day 1	60–135	**Daily Dozen**	12
		Cardiovascular Endurance Moderate intensity (running, biking, hiking, swimming, fast walking, or a combination)	45–120
Day 2	12	**Daily Dozen/Rest**	12
Day 3	50–55	**Circuit Training:**	
		Cardio Warmup: Run or run/walk to location for Basic Circuit	5
		Daily Dozen	12
		Basic Circuit x 3: Perform each of the following exercises for 40 seconds each, with 20 seconds of rest in between. One time through the list of exercises equals one circuit. Do 3 circuits with minimal rest in between circuits: Push-ups, Steam Engines on Back, Squats, Ranger Crawls, Jump Rope or Jumping Jacks, Burpees, Russian Twists, Shuttle Run	25
		Home Stretch	10
Day 4	55–85	**Daily Dozen**	12
		Tempo Workout: Choose a cardio activity you enjoy, such as running, fast walking, cycling, or swimming. For your Tempo Workout, do the following: **Warm Up**—10 minutes at an easy pace (around 50% of your maximum effort).	30–60

WEEK 5	TOTAL MINUTES	EXERCISE AND INTENSITY	MINUTES PER ROUTINE
		Tempo—Speed up your pace so that you are closer to 70% to 80% of your maximum effort. *Duration: Beginners—10 minutes Intermediate—20 minutes Advanced—30 minutes*	
		Cool Down—10 minutes at an easy pace	
		Or Cross Train: Daily Dozen plus 2 minutes of cardio exercise between each routine (running, jumping rope, jumping jacks, fast walking, run/walk, or similar)	
		Home Stretch	10
DAY 5	50–55	**Circuit Training:**	
		Cardio Warmup: Run or run/walk to location for Basic Circuit	5
		Daily Dozen	12
		Basic Circuit x 3: Perform each of the following exercises for 40 seconds each, with 20 seconds of rest in between. One time through the list of exercises equals one circuit. Do 3 circuits with minimal rest in between circuits: Push-ups, Steam Engines on Back, Squats, Ranger Crawls, Jump Rope or Jumping Jacks, Burpees, Russian Twists, Shuttle Run	25
		Home Stretch	10
DAY 6	12	**Daily Dozen/Rest**	12
DAY 7	120	**Cornerstone Workout: Perfect Balance**	120

WEEK 5: DAY BY DAY

DAY 1

Start the day with your **Daily Dozen**. For your moderate-intensity **cardiovascular endurance activity,** keep the duration at 45 to 120 minutes, as always making sure to pace yourself and choose a duration that feels right to you.

DAY 2

Start your day with the **Daily Dozen,** and then enjoy a day of **restoration and relaxation.**

understanding proprioception

Say this word five times fast: pro-pri-o-cep-tion. Then try to spell it. Whether that trips you up or not (it tripped us up!), you'll trip less—literally—by working on your balance as part of your outdoor fitness journey. That's because outdoor exercise increases our proprioception—the ability to sense our surroundings even when our usual senses (such as sight) are compromised. How do you keep from falling when walking through a darkened room? How can you stand up when your eyes are closed? The ability to sense where your body is in relation to your surroundings is the key to proprioception, and it improves markedly with outdoor exercise. In the outdoors, every time you move, your surroundings change. That makes demands on our brains and bodies to take in new information about our surroundings so that without even sensing it, we constantly improve our ability to balance. Enjoy watching the trees pass as you run from one exercise location to the next...or the reflections coming off water if you're exercising near a lake...or the movements of the people around you. You're improving your proprioception with every move you make outdoors. Your commitment so far is a strong indicator of your success to come.

DAY 3

Same as last week: your Basic Circuit workout. **Run for 5 minutes** to a location for your circuit, perform your **Daily Dozen,** and then perform 3 rounds of the **Basic Circuit** (see the workout chart above for the exercise list). Finish with your **Home Stretch.** Set aside around 1 hour for this workout.

DAY 4

Challenge by Choice: Schedule an hour today for either a Tempo Workout or your usual outdoor Cross-Training Workout. You have choices for your **Cross-Training Workout:** you could do the same workout you've done so far in this program, or for variety, take one of the Cornerstone Workouts you've done and simply cut it in half, so that you're working out for an hour or so. If you prefer a **Tempo Workout** this week, choose the challenge that's right for you. Start with a warmup at moderate intensity (50 percent of your maximum effort), and then push your pace up to 70 or 80 percent of your maximum effort. Do this for 10 minutes if you're a beginner, 20 if you're an intermediate athlete, and 30 minutes if you're advanced. While you should not feel out of breath, you should feel as though this is a significant effort that requires concentration. (See the sidebar "Endurance Cross-Training: Inspiration," in Week 2, for more infomation about how to gauge the intensity of your workouts.) Finish with 10 minutes at an easy pace, and top it off with your **Home Stretch**.

DAY 5

Same as Day 3: the Basic Circuit workout. **Run for 5 minutes** to a location for your circuit, perform your **Daily Dozen,** and then perform 3 rounds of the **Basic Circuit** (see the workout chart above for the exercise list). Finish with your **Home Stretch.**

DAY 6

Start your day with the **Daily Dozen**. For the rest of the day, give your body some well-deserved **restoration and relaxation**.

DAY 7

Time for your **Perfect Balance Cornerstone Workout.**

PERFECT BALANCE: THE CORNERSTONE WORKOUT

You've been doing balance exercises since Week 1. They're such an integral part of the program because they inform everything we do. Balance involves any exercise that requires you to stand on one leg. In other words, you're doing balance exercises every time you walk. The purpose of this workout week is not to spend all of our time balancing on one leg, but to add specific exercises designed to challenge balance and stability. There is a particular focus on muscle groups required to both remain in static balanced positions (standing on one leg) and muscles that must remain stable in moving balance situations (running around a corner or on uneven terrain).

perfect balance: inspiration

How relevant is balance to the outdoor athlete? Anyone who has climbed a mountain or stepped into a boat will know the importance of balance. The subtleties of balance also have a dramatic effect on things we take for granted, like turning a corner on a bicycle, changing direction while we run, running across a tennis court to hit a ball, or playing catch with a child. Balance is integral to every motion our bodies make on a daily basis. Balance speaks to where you are in space at all times. And while it's true one needs a high level of balance to perform an intricate yoga pose, that's no less than is required for skiing, snowboarding, ice skating, or for that matter, an Olympic long jumper launching into the air, about to make contact with a sand pit.

This workout will put you in touch with your sense of balance—and you may discover that it needs work. Have confidence going into this week that the exercises will improve both your static and moving balance. When we build these exercises into our regular workout, we will run better, climb better, ride better, ski better—in other words, we'll be able to *live* better.

GEAR LIST

▪ Your usual kit: a sports watch, water, energy snack, small notebook and pen, first-aid kit, cell phone, and sun protection if necessary.
▪ A 10-yard length of rope (or your 20-yard rope with 10 yards marked on it).
▪ Eight cones, rocks, or other markers for marking exercise stations (optional).

IDEAL TERRAIN

▪ A log, bench, or other raised platform for One-Legged Squats. To be sure it will give you adequate support, test it first: it should be high enough so that when you do a regular two-legged Squat, at the lowest position, your bottom should just touch the log or bench.
Note: At many parks you can find a long row of logs sitting end to end marking trails. You can use them both for Squats and other balance exercises such as a balance walk or balance push-out, using the logs as a natural balance beam.
▪ A sand pit or grassy space for balance exercises.
▪ A beach or grassy area for rope drills.
▪ A place where you can tie your 10-yard length of rope between two trees, park benches, railings, or other objects.

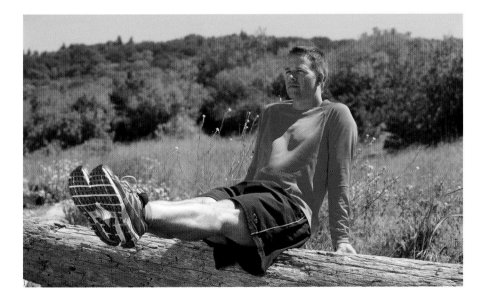

THE EXERCISES:

- For the Daily Dozen exercises, turn to page 67.
- For the Home Stretch exercises, turn to page 75.
- For all other exercises, turn to Appendix A, "Compendium of Exercises," page 223.

PERFECT BALANCE: MINUTE BY MINUTE

00:00 to 00:20

We'll do our usual **warmup** this week: 10 minutes of **running or a walk/run,** followed by the **Daily Dozen.** Throw in an additional challenge this week: try doing the exercises with your eyes closed for everything except the Lunges (where you need to see where you are stepping).

00:20 to 00:25

Run or run/walk for 5 minutes to a bench, log, or other raised platform. Here we'll do One-Legged Squats—10 reps on each leg.

00:25 to 00:35

Next, **run or run/walk** to a sand pit or a grassy field for the following set of **balance exercises.**

- Vector Toe Touches—10 reps
- Side to Side Hops—6 reps on two legs; then 3 each on single leg
- Backwards Lunge to High Knee—10 reps
- Lawnmower Pulls—5 reps on each leg
- Thirsty Bird—10 reps

00:35 to 01:00

Run for 10 minutes. You'll be heading for a beach or a grassy area where you'll do a series of **rope drills.**

Lay the rope on the ground. Walk along the rope, touching toe to heel with each step, one time up and down the rope.

Next, start with your toes touching the rope, and walk by touching feet side to side. Walk this way one time up and down the rope.

On the third time, try a zigzag jump: jump with feet together back and forth across the rope, going up and down the length of the rope. Finally,

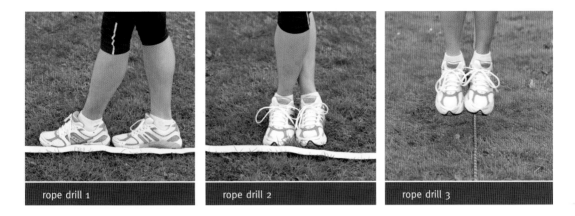

rope drill 1   rope drill 2   rope drill 3

repeat the first two exercises with your hands behind your back for an added balance challenge.

Next, tie the rope 6 inches off the ground between two trees, railings, or park benches. Step over the rope, one foot after the other, in a zigzag pattern, all the way up and back over the length of the rope. (If you can't find a place to tie the rope above the ground, you can do this exercise by making an exaggerated high stepping movement as you step over the rope on the ground.)

Next, come back to your starting point. This time, really engage the heel as you high-step. The heel should touch the ground on every step this time. Step in a zigzag pattern up and down the length of the rope.

Finally, come back to your starting point and do the heel-focused step sequence one more time, with one modification: keep your hands behind your back at all times.

01:00 to 01:10

Eyes-closed walking drill. Set 2 cones about 3 feet apart on the ground. Create a lane about 15 yards long by lining up 6 additional cones about 5 yards apart behind the first 2 cones. Walk from one end of the lane to the other, eyes closed, trying not to touch the cones on either side or to step out of bounds. If you're doing this exercise with a partner, see who can go all the way to the end of the lane first without stepping outside the cones.

01:10 to 01:20

Next, we'll do **one-legged balance exercises**. Start by standing on one leg,

why are my eyes closed?

A lot of people freeze up at first when looking at performing a task like the eyes-closed walking drill. But it's a big confidence-builder. It forces you to confront the question: what do you do when you lose one of the key ingredients to good balance—your sight? You may know someone who is visually impaired who moves with great confidence and sureness—that's evidence of how strongly they have compensated for the loss of sight with other faculties related to balance. The goal of this exercise is to improve your balance by taking away one of those balance-related faculties. It's a great exercise to do with others, especially because your workout partners can keep an eye on you to make sure you don't stray from the cone lane, fall, or stumble.

the standing leg strong, knee unbent, for as long as you can. Time yourself with a sports watch. If you last for 10 seconds or less, you'll see fast improvement as you train your balance more often. Thirty seconds is excellent, and a challenge for most people. One minute is a fantastic time. Believe it or not, we've had adventX athletes last for up to 3 minutes, but that's extremely rare. Wherever you find yourself, know that you will improve in time. After you've done the one-leg balance exercise once on each leg, repeat with your eyes closed to add an extra challenge.

🕐 **01:20 to 01:30**
Next, we'll do a **circuit of exercises for core strength**—a key set of muscles to strengthen for improved balance. Perform 10 repetitions of each exercise in succession with no rest in between, staying in the same location:

▪ Steam Engines on Back
▪ Mountain Climbers
▪ Push-outs
▪ Ranger Crawls
▪ Russian Twists

- Side Planks (hold each side for 30 seconds)
- Donkey Kicks
- Dolphins
- Crocodiles
- Scissors

01:30 to 01:40
Run or run/walk for 10 minutes to the location for your Home Stretch.

01:40 to 01:50
Home Stretch. And you're done—congratulations.

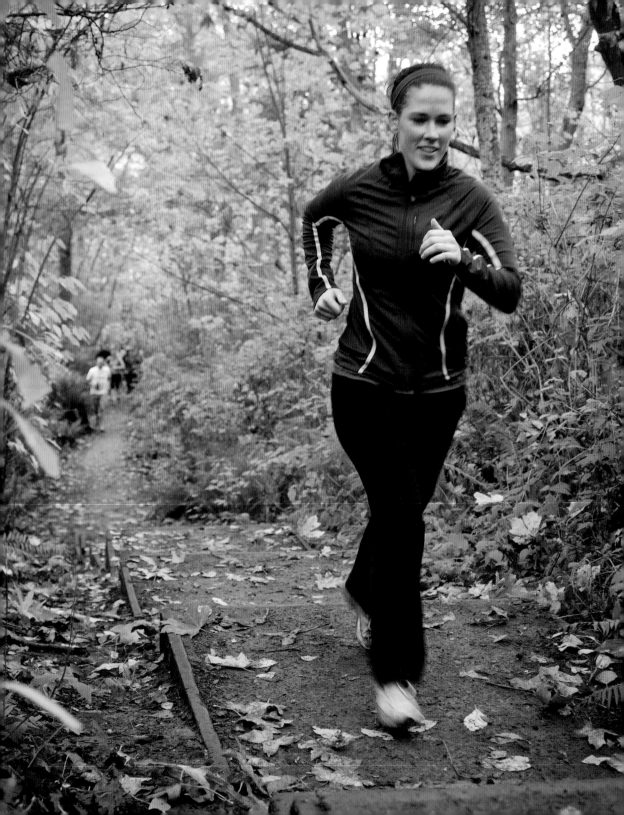

week 6 elevation

**Ready to go up, up, and away? You will be after a week of great condition-
ing workouts and a demanding, hill-based Cornerstone Workout designed to
bring both your strength and endurance to new heights.**

WEEK 6: FIRST NOTES

This week we'll explore going up via hills or staircases—whatever you have
available in your workout area. In Seattle, long staircases are everywhere,
linking streets in hilly neighborhoods throughout the city. Our athletes use
them as one of the natural training tools we find in our area—and training hills and stairs helps you to develop excellent core strength and muscle
endurance. I feel so strongly about the return on investment you'll get from
stair and hill climbing that I've devoted an entire workout to it. Once you
give it a try, I think you'll be hooked as well.

WEEK 6: WORKOUT CHART

WEEK 6	TOTAL MINUTES	EXERCISE AND INTENSITY	MINUTES PER ROUTINE
Day 1	60–135	**Daily Dozen**	12
		Cardiovascular Endurance Moderate intensity (running, biking, hiking, swimming, fast walking, or a combination)	45–120
Day 2	12	**Daily Dozen/Rest**	12
Day 3	50–55	**Circuit Training:**	
		Cardio Warmup: Run or run/walk to location for Basic Circuit	5
		Daily Dozen	12
		Basic Circuit x 3: Perform each of the following exercises for 40 seconds each, with 20 seconds of rest in between. One time through the list of exercises equals one circuit. Do 3 circuits with minimal rest in between circuits: Push-ups, Steam Engines on Back, Squats, Ranger Crawls, Jump Rope or Jumping Jacks, Burpees, Russian Twists, Shuttle Run	25
		Home Stretch	10
Day 4	55–85	**Daily Dozen**	12
		Tempo Workout: Choose a cardio activity you enjoy, such as running, fast walking, cycling, or swimming.	30–60
		For your Tempo Workout, do the following: **Warm Up**—10 minutes at an easy pace (around 50% of your maximum effort).	

WEEK 6	TOTAL MINUTES	EXERCISE AND INTENSITY	MINUTES PER ROUTINE
		Tempo—Speed up your pace so that you are closer to 70% to 80% of your maximum effort. *Duration: Beginners—10 minutes Intermediate—20 minutes Advanced—30 minutes*	
		Cool Down—10 minutes at an easy pace	
		Or Cross Train: Daily Dozen plus 2 minutes of cardio exercise between each routine (running, jumping rope, jumping jacks, fast walking, run/walk, or similar)	
		Home Stretch	10
DAY 5	50–55	**Circuit Training:**	
		Cardio Warmup: Run or run/walk to location for Basic Circuit	5
		Daily Dozen	12
		Basic Circuit x 3: Perform each of the following exercises for 40 seconds each, with 20 seconds of rest in between. One time through the list of exercises equals one circuit. Do 3 circuits with minimal rest in between circuits: Push-ups, Steam Engines on Back, Squats, Ranger Crawls, Jump Rope or Jumping Jacks, Burpees, Russian Twists, Shuttle Run	25
		Home Stretch	10
DAY 6	12	**Daily Dozen/Rest**	12
DAY 7	120	**Cornerstone Workout: Elevation**	120

WEEK 6: DAY BY DAY

DAY 1

Start the day with your **Daily Dozen**. For the moderate-intensity **cardiovascular endurance activity,** keep your duration at 45 to 120 minutes, as always making sure to pace yourself and choose a duration that feels right to you.

DAY 2

Start your day with the **Daily Dozen,** and then enjoy a day of **restoration and relaxation.**

DAY 3

Same as last week: your Basic Circuit workout. **Run for 5 minutes** to a location for your circuit, perform your **Daily Dozen,** and then perform 3 rounds of the **Basic Circuit** (see the workout chart above for the exercise list). Finish with your **Home Stretch.** Set aside around an hour for this workout.

DAY 4

Challenge by Choice: schedule an hour today for either a Tempo Workout or your usual outdoor Cross-Training Workout. For your **Cross-Training Workout,** you can either do the same workout you've done so far in this program, or as in previous weeks, take one of the Cornerstone Workouts you've done so far and cut it in half. For a **Tempo Workout,** choose the challenge that's right for you: after warming up at moderate intensity for 10 minutes, push your pace: 10 minutes for beginners, 20 for intermediate athletes, and 30 minutes for advanced athletes. Finish with 10 minutes at an easy pace, and top it off with your **Home Stretch.**

DAY 5

Same as Day 3: the Basic Circuit workout. **Run for 5 minutes** to a location for your circuit, perform your **Daily Dozen,** and then perform 3 rounds of the **Basic Circuit** (see the workout chart above for the exercise list). Finish with your **Home Stretch.**

DAY 6

Start your day with the **Daily Dozen**. For the rest of the day, give your body some well-deserved **restoration and relaxation.**

DAY 7

Time for your **Elevation Cornerstone Workout**. Details below.

ELEVATION: THE CORNERSTONE WORKOUT

The first consideration for the elevation workout is to find a place where you can do it. Many cities have parks with hills. You're looking for options: perhaps a local stadium with lots of stairs, or in a pinch, a tall stairwell inside a building. For this class, identify two types of hills or stairs for your workout— a short set of stairs or hill, and a longer set of stairs or hill.

There are a few secrets to getting the best stair workout for your body. This is a place where borrowing techniques from mountain climbers can assist us. Climbers use two different styles: the simplest and fastest method to use for a short period of time is to climb as if you are running, pushing off the ground from the balls of your feet, using your arms for propulsion. However, this method is only effective for a few minutes, since it tends to put significant stress on the front of the body (the shins and quadriceps in particular), as well as the calves, since you're standing on the balls of your feet.

The second technique is a mountain step, also known in mountaineering parlance as the *rest step*. When you're climbing for a much longer period of time, the rest step will allow your leg muscles to recover in between so you can keep going without getting fatigued. The rest step specifically targets the power muscles of the lower core, namely your glutes, hamstrings, and deep abdominal and back muscles. Not only does it firm up your behind, it also improves your posture. Here's how to do it:

Approach the steps or hill with your shoulders and hips square, in the direction you're going to ascend. Get close to the first step, lift one leg up onto the first step, and pause. The pause is the key to this step. At this point, all of your weight is on your back leg. Your front leg has no tension, and you'll feel the hamstrings and glutes engaged.

Next, quickly transfer your weight to the front foot as you push down, drive the energy down through your heel, and quickly bring the rear leg into the "up" position—stepping forward onto the next step—and then pause. Now your weight will be on your back leg. This takes a little bit of practice; to perfect the step, go a little slower at first, concentrating on keeping the weight on your back leg and the force being driven through the heel as you push up using glutes and hamstrings.

Focus on your heel engaging every time you take a step, wherever you go—in your house, getting into your car, or even walking around in your office. When your weight is on your heel, the power muscles (gluteus maximus and hamstrings) are engaged. Another benefit is less stress on the quads and the front of the legs, which appears to have a positive effect in avoiding knee pain and overuse injuries.

GEAR LIST
∎ Your usual kit: a sports watch, water, energy snack, small notebook and pen, first-aid kit, cell phone, and sun protection if necessary.

IDEAL TERRAIN
∎ A grassy field for your warmup.
∎ One shorter and one longer hill or staircase.
   Note: The shorter hill or staircase should be something you can ascend at a moderately quick pace in 45 to 90 seconds. The longer hill should be

elevation: inspiration

There are many ways to "elevate" your training. One method is to do exactly what we're going to do in this week's Cornerstone Workout: utilize hills, stairs, and other natural tools for propelling our bodies upward. There's another, more metaphorical way to think of elevation, and that's in the kinds of goals you set for yourself, whether for this workout in particular, this workout week, or this entire season. You've reached Week 6 of your season—an important milestone. You're halfway through. Check in with yourself—have your goals changed? Are you starting to dream of bigger things? Pay attention to where your thoughts are this week as you lock in on your goals—you can elevate those to match your new fitness level just as much as you can physically elevate your body in this week's Cornerstone Workout.

something that takes 6 to 10 minutes to climb. In a pinch, you can create the larger hill by simply going up and down the shorter hill multiple times. An ideal hill is steep enough that it would be a challenge to run the whole way (unless you're an expert trail runner). Use your own judgment to find the hill that feels right for your workout.

THE EXERCISES:

- For the Daily Dozen exercises, turn to page 67.
- For the Home Stretch exercises, turn to page 75.
- For all other exercises, turn to Appendix A, "Compendium of Exercises," page 223.

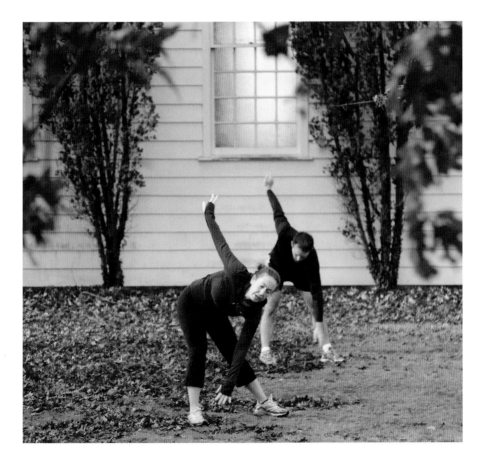

ELEVATION: MINUTE BY MINUTE

 00:00 to 00:20
Easy run or **run/walk for 10 minutes** to your warmup location. Do your **Daily Dozen** here.

 00:20 to 00:35
Once you're done with the Daily Dozen, **walk or run lightly** to your shorter hill or staircase. Your first stair workout is a simple one: **walk up and down the stairs** at a moderate pace for 10 minutes. (If that sounds easy, ask yourself whether it's easy after 7 minutes or so have elapsed.)

 00:35 to 00:55
Now, **run or run/walk for 5 to 10 minutes** to a grassy field or other flat area with a soft surface for a **core exercise circuit**. Do each of the following exercises for 10 reps each, and perform the entire circuit 2 times. Take 10 seconds of rest in between each exercise in the first circuit, and just 2 seconds between each exercise in the second circuit. This is a Challenge by Choice moment— a challenging set of exercises for your lower core and back, so remember to emphasize good form on these movements. These exercises can all be performed in one location, so there is no need to set up cones for this circuit.

- Crocodiles
- Scissors
- Steam Engines on Back
- Russian Twists
- Push-outs

 00:55 to 01:15
From here, **run another 5 to 10 minutes**—either out and back to the same grassy space, or to another space nearer to the bigger of the two hills you've chosen for this workout. You've likely forgotten about the stairs by now— your core should feel strong after the core exercise circuit. Now take the next step—an **upper body circuit.** As with the previous core circuit, do 10 reps of each exercise and two full circuits, with 10 seconds of rest between exercises in the first circuit, and two seconds in the second circuit. Your goal here is to get through the entire circuit twice using excellent workout form. As with the core exercises, these can be done in one place—no need to set up cones for this circuit.

- Seagulls
- Triceps Dips
- Push-ups
- Wide-Arm Push-ups
- Diamond Push-ups

A note on Push-ups: Push-ups are an incredibly important exercise. Don't be concerned if you still feel as though you can't do the full movement with your knees off the ground. For these Push-ups, you can perform them against a wall to lower the resistance so that you can concentrate on completing the movement with good form. Your arms will certainly feel the work and you'll sense a good burn, but it shouldn't be any more uncomfortable than your abs or legs felt when you focused on them.

01:15 to 01:40
Now it's time to find your big hill. **Run or run/walk for 10 minutes** to get to the bottom of your hill or staircase. Your goal here is to **walk vigorously uphill 1 or 2 times,** depending on how you feel. (Wait until you've completed one hill climb before you decide whether to do a second one.) Remember this adage: "With hills, it's pace that kills." In other words, it's not about the elevation. If you find your correct pace, you can climb all day, but if you go too fast, you won't last more than a few minutes. Go slower than you think you want to, but finish quickly in the last minutes. By the top of the hill you should be sweating and breathing hard, and you should feel out of breath, with no interest in striking up a conversation with the person next to you! Focus on one thing: getting to the top. When you do reach the top, don't stop there; keep walking for another minute or two, just to let your body relax and your heart rate come back down.

01:40 to 01:50
A **short recovery workout** of about 10 minutes is designed to rebalance ourselves and recalibrate our bodies with big movements, taking us through a full range of motion in all of our body's axes.
- Squat and Reach
- Twisters
- Arm Circles
- Jog in place for 30 seconds

- Jumping Jacks
- Arm Extenders
- Sumo Squats
- Arm Circles—10 backwards, 10 forwards
- Sun Gods—Do each move for 20 to 30 seconds (Arm Circles to sides, front, and above)

01:50 to 02:05

Take 5 minutes to warm down with an **easy run or run/walk**. Finish up with your **Home Stretch**, taking particular care to stretch your calves and hamstrings. You may want to do the calf and hamstring stretches twice at the end of this class, given the sheer amount of effort those muscles were required to put forth for the elevation workout.

more thoughts on elevation

The primary purpose of this workout is to build muscle endurance, but there is a secondary goal: anaerobic cardiovascular development, or the ability to push hard for a short period of time. You'll notice both your overall endurance and the strength required for short, hard bursts of effort improving as you do more stair and hill workouts.

Compared to other types of workouts, stairs and hills offer significant gains in a short period of time. That's largely due to the considerable energy expenditure and high output of power required to move the body uphill against gravity. Moving away from the earth is always a tough order—it's pretty difficult to get away from gravitational pull.

We don't necessarily think of gravity being a factor when we're working out in the outdoors, but in fact it's one of the natural phenomena and the primary factor in creating resistance in all body weight exercises. So consider the power of the earth's gravitational pull as you work up to doing harder and harder stair workouts, and appreciate how much the natural world has given you to work with on your fitness journey.

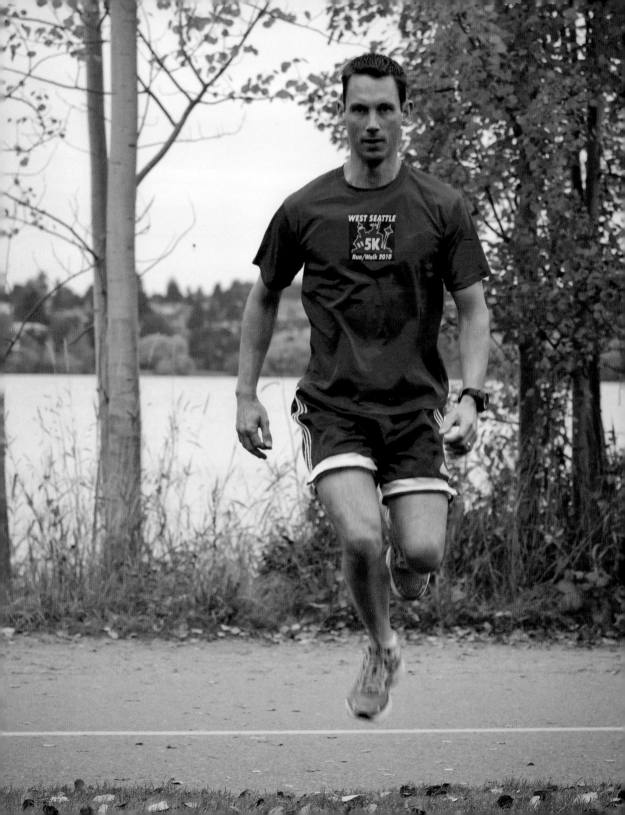

week 7 el rapido

This is the week where we need some speed! After a week of conditioning workouts, sprints and quick exercise circuits in your Cornerstone Workout will maximize your speed while injecting a healthy dose of fun into your routine.

WEEK 7: FIRST NOTES

This week presents a big challenge. It's a time where you can choose to increase endurance with a longer Cardiovascular Endurance Workout than you've done yet. It's also an opportunity to do another Tempo Workout (or your first one, if you haven't yet tried that challenge), and a chance to try out our "El Rapido" Cornerstone Workout. You'll build quickness in your step, your body's movements, and your reaction time. We'll also work on developing pure speed—all skills that will make you a faster, snappier, and more well-rounded athlete.

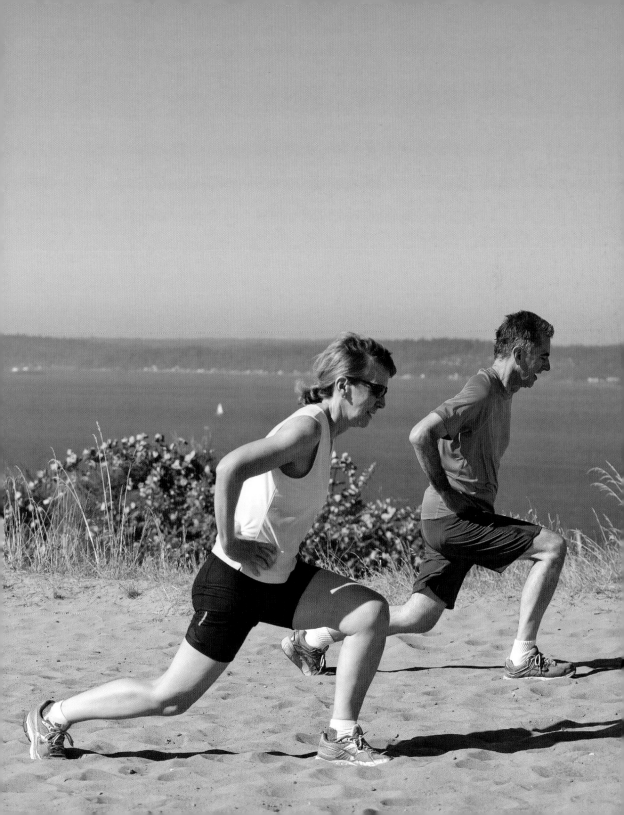

WEEK 7: WORKOUT CHART

WEEK 7	TOTAL MINUTES	EXERCISE AND INTENSITY	MINUTES PER ROUTINE
Day 1	60–135	**Daily Dozen**	12
		Cardiovascular Endurance Moderate intensity (running, biking, hiking, swimming, fast walking, or a combination)	45–120
Day 2	12	**Daily Dozen/Rest**	12
Day 3	50–55	**Circuit Training:**	
		Cardio Warmup: Run or run/walk to location for Basic Circuit	5
		Daily Dozen	12
		Basic Circuit x 3: Perform each of the following exercises for 40 seconds each, with 20 seconds of rest in between. One time through the list of exercises equals one circuit. Do 3 circuits with minimal rest in between circuits: Push-ups, Steam Engines on Back, Squats, Ranger Crawls, Jump Rope or Jumping Jacks, Burpees, Russian Twists, Shuttle Run	25
		Home Stretch	10
Day 4	55–85	**Daily Dozen**	12
		Tempo Workout: Choose a cardio activity you enjoy, such as running, fast walking, cycling, or swimming. For your Tempo Workout, do the following: **Warm Up**—10 minutes at an easy pace (around 50% of your maximum effort).	30–60

WEEK 7	TOTAL MINUTES	EXERCISE AND INTENSITY	MINUTES PER ROUTINE
		Tempo—Speed up your pace so that you are closer to 70% to 80% of your maximum effort. *Duration: Beginners—10 minutes Intermediate—20 minutes Advanced—30 minutes*	
		Cool Down—10 minutes at an easy pace	
		Or Cross Train: Daily Dozen plus 2 minutes of cardio exercise between each routine (running, jumping rope, jumping jacks, fast walking, run/walk, or similar)	
		Home Stretch	10
DAY 5	50–55	**Circuit Training:**	
		Cardio Warmup: Run or run/walk to location for Basic Circuit	5
		Daily Dozen	12
		Basic Circuit x 3: Perform each of the following exercises for 40 seconds each, with 20 seconds of rest in between. One time through the list of exercises equals one circuit. Do 3 circuits with minimal rest in between circuits: Push-ups, Steam Engines on Back, Squats, Ranger Crawls, Jump Rope or Jumping Jacks, Burpees, Russian Twists, Shuttle Run	25
		Home Stretch	10
DAY 6	12	**Daily Dozen/Rest**	12
DAY 7	120	**Cornerstone Workout: El Rapido**	120

WEEK 7: DAY BY DAY

DAY 1
Start with your **Daily Dozen**. For your moderate-intensity **cardiovascular endurance activity,** keep your duration at 45 to 120 minutes and pace yourself moderately. Choose a duration that feels right to you, perhaps increasing it by a few minutes over last week's time if you're so inclined.

DAY 2
Start your day with the **Daily Dozen,** and then enjoy a day of **restoration and relaxation**.

DAY 3
You know the routine: this is your Basic Circuit workout day. Set aside around 1 hour for this workout. **Run for 5 minutes** to a location for your circuit, perform your **Daily Dozen,** and then perform three rounds of the **Basic Circuit** (see the workout chart for the exercise list). Finish with your **Home Stretch.**

DAY 4
Challenge by Choice: schedule an hour today for either a Tempo Workout or your usual outdoor Cross-Training Workout. You have choices for your **Cross-Training Workout:** do the same workout you've done so far in this program, or for variety, take one of the Cornerstone Workouts you've done so far, and simply cut it in half so that you're working out for an hour or so. If you haven't tried the **Tempo Workout** yet, let this week be your opportunity: warm up at moderate intensity for 10 minutes, and then push the pace with your desired cardio activity: 10 minutes for beginners, 20 for intermediate athletes, and 30 minutes for advanced athletes, going at around 70 percent to 80 percent of maximum effort. Finish with 10 minutes at an easy pace to cool down, and top it off with your **Home Stretch.**

DAY 5
Same as Day 3: your Basic Circuit workout. **Run for 5 minutes** to a location for your circuit, perform your **Daily Dozen,** and then perform 3 rounds of the **Basic Circuit** (see the workout chart for the exercise list). Finish with your **Home Stretch.**

el rapido: inspiration

Everyone can get faster, and it's not as difficult as most people think. Ask ten people how to run faster and the answers will mostly consist of people saying that you have to try harder. As in many aspects of life, it's not about trying harder, it's about being more skillful and more efficient. The El Rapido workout is designed to help you move more efficiently. The design of the El Rapido workout is to warm you up and to challenge you in ways that create an environment where you can move more quickly.

DAY 6
Start your day with the **Daily Dozen**. For the rest of the day, enjoy a time of **restoration and relaxation.**

DAY 7
The time has come for your **El Rapido Cornerstone Workout**. Prepare for a great ride—your workout details are below.

EL RAPIDO: THE CORNERSTONE WORKOUT

GEAR LIST
▪ Your usual kit: a sports watch, water, energy snack, small notebook and pen, first-aid kit, cell phone, and sun protection if necessary.
▪ Nine cones or rocks to set up the Cone Drill and the Illinois Agility Drill.
▪ Long measuring tape to set distances for the Cone Drill and the Illinois Agility Drill. You can estimate the distances if you don't have a measuring tape available.
▪ Jump rope (optional).

IDEAL TERRAIN
▪ A grassy field for your Daily Dozen and other warmup exercises.

> ▪ A sand pit or hard-packed beach if possible; otherwise, a grassy field for the X Agility Drill.
> ▪ Your timed-run course.
> ▪ A baseball diamond or grassy field for the Cal Ripken Special.

THE EXERCISES:
> ▪ For the Daily Dozen exercises, turn to page 67.
> ▪ For the Home Stretch exercises, turn to page 75.
> ▪ For all other exercises, turn to Appendix A, "Compendium of Exercises," page 223.

EL RAPIDO: MINUTE BY MINUTE

00:00 to 00:20
Start with your normal warmup—5 to 10 minutes of **light running** or a run/walk to a grassy field, followed by the **Daily Dozen**.

00:20 to 00:40
Now, do a more advanced warmup for your lower legs and core muscles as preparation for the harder work to come. **Perform 10 reps** of each exercise:
▪ Leg Swings
▪ Ankle Alphabet
▪ Backward and Forward Walking

Next, to warm up the lower core (quads, hamstrings, glutes, and iliotibial bands), do a more vigorous series. **Perform 10 reps** of each exercise:
▪ Squats
▪ Lunges
▪ Side Lunges
▪ Clock Lunges

We'll continue with more overall warmup exercises for your core and upper body—perform, you guessed it, **10 reps** per exercise:
▪ Squats (yes, another set!)
▪ Power Jumps
▪ Jump Rope or Jumping Jacks—1 minute

- Scissor Jumps
- Crocodiles
- Scissors
- Push-ups
- Plank
- Arm Extenders
- Arm Chops
- Seagulls
- Arm Circles
- Accelerating Arms

🕐 **00:40 to 00:50**
Now, we'll do a series of **agility drills**.

X Agility Drill. Draw two intersecting lines in the sand, about 6 feet long, in the shape of a cross (+) in a sand pit or on a beach. (If you don't have access to a sand pit or a beach, you can use sticks or twigs to mark the ground, or just make a mental note of where the lines would be drawn on the ground.) For the first part of the drill, jump from side to side, left to right, in the top half of the cross, for 10 reps back and forth. Then, jump back and forth, top to bottom, on the left side of the cross, for 10 reps. Finally, jump in a diagonal motion—top left to bottom right, to bottom left, to top right, to top left, for 10 reps.

Cone Drill. Place five cones in a straight row, spacing them a couple feet apart so the entire row is about 9 feet long. Three feet away from the first row, set up a row of four cones, staggering them between the first five cones (see illustration). Starting at the cone in the lower left of the illustration, run in a zigzag fashion around each cone in the lower row up to and around each cone in the upper row. When you reach the end of the bottom row, run straight up past the top row, turn to run the length of the rows, and then turn again to return to your starting point.

Illinois Agility Drill. (See sidebar on next page for setup instructions.) Perform the drill once for practice, rest for a minute, and then do it again for time, recording your score in your notebook.

the illinois agility drill

Agility is defined as the ability to change direction easily. The drills included in this week's Cornerstone Workout will develop that exact skill. By far the most fun—and most challenging to set up—will be the Illinois Agility Drill (also known as the Illinois Agility Test). To set up the course, place eight cones or rocks in the following pattern:

Place four cones or rocks in a square, one cone at each corner. The square should be about 10 yards by 6 yards (30 feet by 18 feet). Place the remaining four cones down the center of the square, equally spaced apart. In order to make it the entire 10 yards, the cones will be about 3 feet apart.

To perform the drill, start at the cone in the lower left-hand corner of the illustration. Sprint to the lower right-hand corner cone and then back toward the starting cone. Next, run in a zigzag style through the middle cones and back. Finally, sprint to the upper right-hand corner cone and then back to the upper left-hand corner cone.

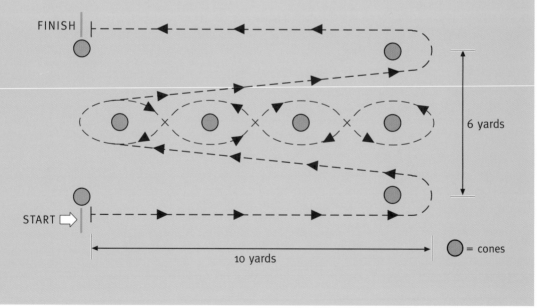

The Cone Drill Setup

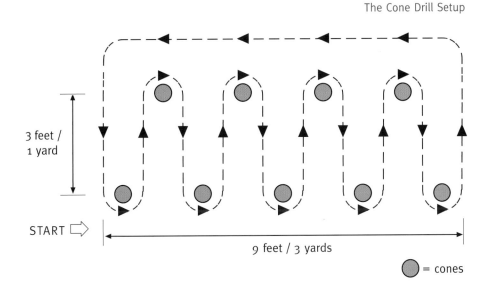

3 feet / 1 yard

START ⟹

9 feet / 3 yards

⬤ = cones

After these cone drills, prepare to run by performing the following warmups specific to running. Perform each warmup for 30 seconds:
▮ Butt Kicks
▮ Gazelles

Run for about 5 to 10 minutes at an easy pace to get to the start of your usual timed-run path.

 00:50 to 01:00
Your **timed run.** Be sure to keep track of your time from week to week—you should see yourself slowly starting to improve.

01:00 to 01:10
Next, we'll work on **core training**. Find a place with a picnic bench, log, or stairs—you're looking for a platform to use for Triceps Dips. You can also do your Triceps Dips on the ground if no platform is available. Perform the **10 exercises** listed on the next page for core strength (10 reps per exercise).

explosiveness

There is a lot of explosiveness in this workout. We're developing the anaerobic energy system of the body: the all-out sprint-style work that should leave you gasping for breath. (Contrast that with the aerobic energy system, which does the opposite.) Because this workout trains quickness, you're apt to get tired sooner if you're doing it well, so when we teach this class at adventX, it often becomes closer to a 90-minute workout than a full 2 hours—and we know we've earned it. Give yourself that same treat—work out hard, do everything your body can do for today, and then enjoy the shorter workout day and the longer recovery.

- Crocodiles
- Squat Thrusters
- Burpees
- Triceps Dips
- Push-ups
- Steam Engines on Back
- Mountain Climbers
- Dolphins
- Scissors
- Russian Twists

01:10 to 01:25

Next, lightly run for about 5 minutes to either a baseball diamond or an open field for the Cal Ripken Special drill (a workout on a baseball diamond). If no baseball diamond is available, you can simply measure out a workout space on a soccer field or other grassy space that would mirror the proportions of a baseball diamond (about 60 feet between bases). If you don't have a field at all but just a strip of ground, you can set up cones in a straight line, about 60 feet apart.

The **Cal Ripken Special** consists of the following exercises:

- Start in the dugout (or next to the home plate or starting area). Do 10 Triceps Dips.
- Run to home base. Do 10 Jumping Jacks.
- Run to first base. Do 10 Push-ups.
- Run back to home base. Run to second base (via first base, like a baseball player), and do 10 Squat Thrusters.
- Run back to home base. Run to third base via first and second bases. At third base, do 10 Power Jumps. Run back to home via second base and first base.
- From home base, sprint through all the bases (first to third) and complete the diamond by sprinting from third base to home.

01:25 to 01:45

TIme to start cooling down. Start with a 5- to 10-minute light run to an open field. Then, it's time for your **Home Stretch**. Congratulations—you've completed El Rapido. Relax, enjoy the rest of the day, and celebrate a job well done.

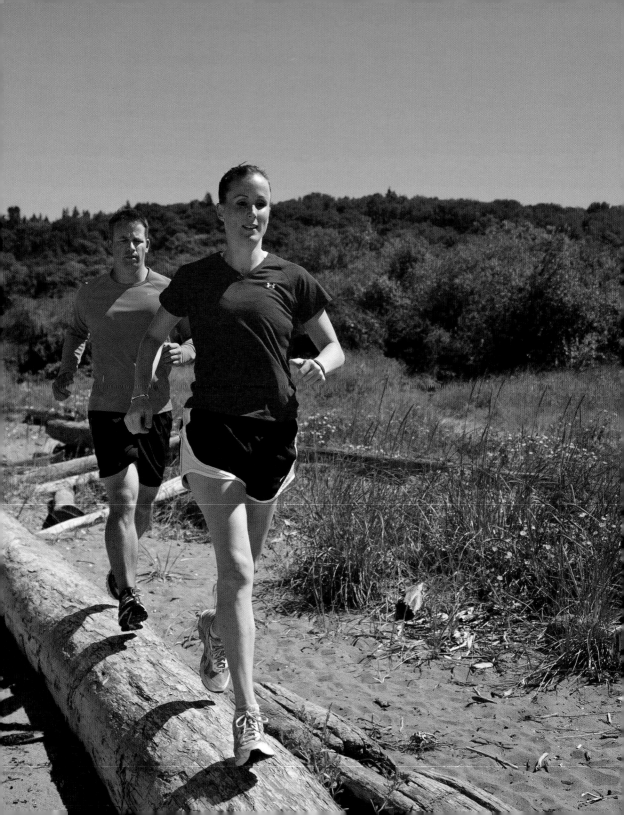

week 8 going long

Weeks 8 through 12 make up the "peaking" cycle of your 12-week workout plan. This week, you'll see options for adding endurance in a few places to your weekly routine. The Going Long Cornerstone Workout will top off the week with an endurance-building regimen that's perfect for anyone training for a longer effort, such as a road race or a long hike. Take this week as an opportunity to get inspired to get even stronger, while dreaming of greater endurance efforts to come.

WEEK 8: FIRST NOTES

From weeks 1 to 3, you were in your **Adaptation** phase: adapting to your new training program. Weeks 4 to 7 were a period of **Building**: adding strength and endurance to your foundation. We've now reached Week 8, the beginning of a 5-week period of **Peaking** your performance. Now we have the option of a longer Cardiovascular Endurance Workout on Day 1—we've moved the upper limit from 120 to 180 minutes. Take the challenge if it appeals to you, and remember to move at moderate intensity at all times.

Most sports or physical activities offer the opportunity to go long—in other words, to cover some serious distance. In a triathlon you can do a sprint race, or you can go long with a full Ironman. Running offers the same thing—a 5K or a full marathon. Cycling, mountain climbing, and other endurance sports all offer their own version of going long. It's a core concept that applies to many sports and other physical activities. This week, take time to notice the physical, mental and emotional transitions you're experiencing as you go from where you are now to the next level of endurance activity.

WEEK 8: WORKOUT CHART

WEEK 8	TOTAL MINUTES	EXERCISE AND INTENSITY	MINUTES PER ROUTINE
Day 1	60–195	**Daily Dozen**	12
		Cardiovascular Endurance Moderate intensity (running, biking, hiking, swimming, fast walking, or a combination)	45–180
Day 2	12	**Daily Dozen/Rest**	12
Day 3	50–55	**Circuit Training:**	
		Cardio Warmup: Run or run/walk to location for Basic Circuit	5
		Daily Dozen	12
		Basic Circuit x 3: Perform each of the following exercises for 40 seconds each, with 20 seconds of rest in between. One time through the list of exercises equals one circuit. Do 3 circuits with minimal rest in between circuits: Push-ups, Steam Engines on Back, Squats, Ranger Crawls, Jump Rope or Jumping Jacks, Burpees, Russian Twists, Shuttle Run	25
		Home Stretch	10
Day 4	55–85	**Daily Dozen**	12
		Tempo Workout: Choose a cardio activity you enjoy, such as running, fast walking, cycling, or swimming. For your Tempo Workout, do the following: **Warm Up**—10 minutes at an easy pace (around 50% of your maximum effort).	30–60

WEEK 8	TOTAL MINUTES	EXERCISE AND INTENSITY	MINUTES PER ROUTINE
		Tempo—Speed up your pace so that you are closer to 70% to 80% of your maximum effort. *Duration: Beginners—10 minutes Intermediate—20 minutes Advanced—30 minutes*	
		Cool Down—10 minutes at an easy pace	
		Or Cross Train: Daily Dozen plus 2 minutes of cardio exercise between each routine (running, jumping rope, jumping jacks, fast walking, run/walk, or similar)	
		Home Stretch	10
DAY 5	50–55	**Circuit Training:**	
		Cardio Warmup: Run or run/walk to location for Basic Circuit	5
		Daily Dozen	12
		Basic Circuit x 3: Perform each of the following exercises for 40 seconds each, with 20 seconds of rest in between. One time through the list of exercises equals one circuit. Do 3 circuits with minimal rest in between circuits: Push-ups, Steam Engines on Back, Squats, Ranger Crawls, Jump Rope or Jumping Jacks, Burpees, Russian Twists, Shuttle Run	25
		Home Stretch	10
DAY 6	12	**Daily Dozen/Rest**	12
DAY 7	120	**Cornerstone Workout: Going Long**	120

WEEK 8: DAY BY DAY

DAY 1

Start the day with your **Daily Dozen**. For your moderate-intensity **cardiovascular endurance activity,** increase the duration if that appeals to you: keep moving from 45 to 180 minutes, whatever feels best for your current level of fitness.

DAY 2

Start your day with the **Daily Dozen,** and then enjoy some **restoration and relaxation.**

DAY 3

Time for your Basic Circuit workout. Set aside around 1 hour for this workout. **Run for 5 minutes** to a location for your circuit, perform your **Daily Dozen,**

going long: inspiration

a short history of long endurance

The long endurance workout has been a staple of Olympic distance runners for half a century. You've likely noticed in the last couple of decades that there has been a strong resurgence of long-distance events in many countries. The number of marathon runners, Ironman competitors, cyclists doing century rides, and multiweek expedition mountain climbers has risen in the past twenty years. We can look to history for other examples of when endurance events were in vogue. In the first half of the twentieth century, there were countless examples of people trying every manner of sports from the sensible to the ridiculous. That included such events as a coast-to-coast running race, where most competitors never got near the finish, to dance marathons and flagpole sitting. Reaching even further back—and further afield—we find examples of athletes undertaking great feats of endurance with not a semblance of the equipment that we possess today.

and then perform 3 rounds of the **Basic Circuit** (see the workout chart for the exercise list). Finish with your **Home Stretch.**

DAY 4

Challenge by Choice: schedule an hour today for either a Tempo Workout or your usual outdoor Cross-Training Workout. As usual, you can choose to do the same **Cross-Training Workout** you've done so far in this program, or perform half of your favorite Cornerstone Workout. If you go for a **Tempo Workout,** remember your guidelines: warm up at moderate intensity for 10 minutes, and then push your pace with your desired cardio activity: 10 minutes for beginners, 20 for intermediate athletes, and 30 minutes for advanced athletes, going at around 70 percent to 80 percent of maximum effort. Finish with 10 minutes at an easy pace to cool down, and top it off with your **Home Stretch**.

DAY 5

Same as Day 3: the Basic Circuit workout. **Run for 5 minutes** to a location for your circuit, perform your **Daily Dozen,** and then perform 3 rounds of the **Basic Circuit** (see the workout chart for the exercise list). Finish with your **Home Stretch.**

DAY 6

Start your day with the **Daily Dozen**. For the rest of the day, enjoy a time of **restoration and relaxation.**

DAY 7

Time for the **Going Long Cornerstone Workout.** Details below.

GOING LONG: THE CORNERSTONE WORKOUT

You'll notice three separate long endurance runs in this workout. If you're not a runner, consider using cycling or swimming as your endurance activity for this workout. You could do your calisthenics at the side of a pool, a lake shore, or just off a bike trail. Use your imagination—the key is to give yourself the opportunity to "go long" by doing just that, using whatever endurance activity you most enjoy. Additionally, you could play around with the prescribed times: the description that follows includes two 20-minute runs and one 30-minute run, but a beginning athlete could do two 10-minute runs and one 20-minute run; for an intermediate athlete it could be 15/15/30; and a more advanced athlete could lengthen the longer run by 10 minutes (for 20/20/40). It's up to you—whatever you feel your body is ready to do is what you should undertake on this day.

GEAR LIST

■ Your usual kit: a sports watch, water, energy snack (especially important today), small notebook and pen, first-aid kit, cell phone, and sun protection if necessary.

IDEAL TERRAIN

■ An area to do an extended run of 20 minutes or so.
■ A grassy field or other soft ground for calisthenics.

THE EXERCISES:

■ For the Daily Dozen exercises, turn to page 67.
■ For the Home Stretch exercises, turn to page 75.
■ For all other exercises, turn to Appendix A, "Compendium of Exercises," page 223.

GOING LONG: MINUTE BY MINUTE

00:00 to 00:20
The usual warmup: **10 minutes of running** or a run/walk to a grassy field for your **Daily Dozen**.

00:20 to 00:40
In this workout, you'll find no major rest periods, nor any super-high-intensity drills or exercises. Instead, today we'll work at a steady, consistent pace, broken up into manageable pieces. The first task of the day is to **run continuously for 20 minutes.** If you're a runner, go at a slow pace; if you're a walker, you may choose to go at a pace faster than your normal walking pace, but one you can sustain for 20 minutes. You also have the option of doing a run/walk, especially if you have struggled with running and long distances in the

prepare and stay safe

Today's workout really starts the day before. All endurance workouts should be fueled with a good meal and good hydration the evening before, but especially those workouts where you sustain hard effort for more than 90 minutes. Also consider your clothing for this workout: comfortable socks will prevent blisters, and weather-appropriate clothing will protect against the elements, whether they be sun, wind, or rain. If it's sunny or rainy, a hat is important. In cooler temperatures, it would be wise to take a light pair of gloves. Much of the challenge involved in training for endurance comes down to protecting yourself against the elements. If you lose too much fluid through sweating, or too much heat through overexposure to cold temperatures or wind, you won't enjoy this workout. Make sure you're well-protected and well-nourished. When you're fueled up and ready to go, you'll find Going Long to be one of your most rewarding weeks in the program.

This workout also gives you the opportunity to experiment with eating and drinking on the run. You don't want to go a whole 2 hours without food or water. Aim to drink 16 ounces of water each hour (more if it's hot outside, or if you're a bigger or taller athlete), and to carry energy gels, bars, or even a bagel to munch on halfway through the workout.

past. If you want to cover long distances, the key will be the run/walk interval. Determining the length of your running and walking intervals is something of an arbitrary decision, but if you're looking for a starting point, try to run for 3 minutes and walk for 2. (See Appendix D for resources on running and incorporating walking breaks into your runs.)

00:40 to 00:50
After the 20-minute run, take **a short rest of a minute or less**. Now, we'll do a **set of calisthenics**, starting at the top of the body and working our way down. Perform one circuit of 10 reps per exercise:

▮ Arm Circles
▮ Push-ups
▮ Triceps Dips
▮ Mountain Climbers

more thoughts on going long

No matter how long you think you can go, you possess more endurance than you can imagine. The key to success in this workout, and in endurance workouts in general, is to break things down into manageable pieces, to get the pace right, to consider the nutritional needs of your body, and to exercise exemplary self-care. You'll notice that there are both long endurance and stationary calisthenics in this workout. The purpose of that switch from covering ground to stationary exercise is to break up the demand on your muscles, ligaments, and tendons that occurs with long endurance efforts, while still maintaining a good level of exertion on the heart and lungs. It bears repeating: pay close attention to intensity. The entire workout should be conducted at a conversational (that is, aerobic) pace. You should feel like you could run or ride alongside a fellow athlete and hold a conversation; in other words, you want to be comfortably below your anaerobic threshold. You should never feel out of breath, and your breathing should never feel heavy or labored.

- Steam Engines on Back
- Side Plank with Arm Reach—10 reps on each side
- Sumo Squats
- Squat Thrusters
- Plank—1 minute (or add a second minute if you're feeling very strong)
- Burpees

 00:50 to 01:10
Take another 1-minute break, and then **repeat the 20-minute run**. Remember to go at a pace you can comfortably sustain for 20 minutes.

 01:10 to 01:20
Next, **repeat the calisthenics circuit** from above.

🕐 **01:20 to 01:50**
Finally, you'll do a **longer run of 30 minutes**. One way to organize this work-out is to do it as an out-and-back course or a loop that gets you back to your warmup location at the end of this run for your Home Stretch. If you've done that, the second 20-minute run would take you to the halfway point of your out-and-back course.

🕐 **01:50 to 02:00**
Home Stretch. You made it—congratulations!

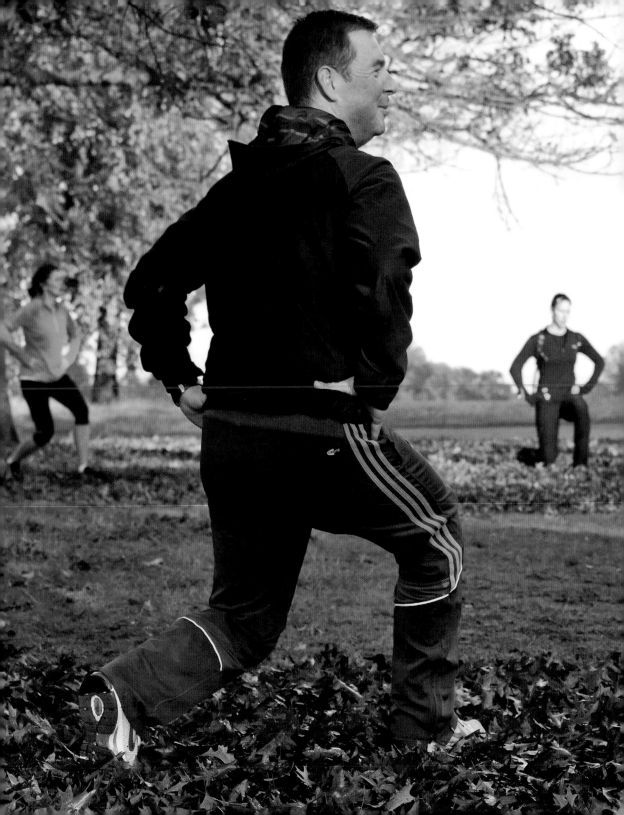

week 9 the one thousand

After another week of conditioning, you'll tackle the One Thousand—a calisthenics workout like no other. We do this workout once a season at adventX to celebrate strength, endurance, and mental toughness. It's great training for getting your mind ready for a long endurance event—no wonder this workout is a favorite with our marathoners and triathletes. Take the challenge!

WEEK 9: FIRST NOTES

Last week we tested endurance by going long. This week, we'll go long in a different way, taxing the muscles through the performance of no less than one thousand repetitions of calisthenics. Strap on your shoes, get your gear, and let's have a great workout and a great celebration of your growing strength and endurance.

WEEK 9: WORKOUT CHART

WEEK 9	TOTAL MINUTES	EXERCISE AND INTENSITY	MINUTES PER ROUTINE
Day 1	60–195	**Daily Dozen**	12
		Cardiovascular Endurance Moderate intensity (running, biking, hiking, swimming, fast walking, or a combination)	45–180
Day 2	12	**Daily Dozen/Rest**	12
Day 3	50–55	**Circuit Training:**	
		Cardio Warmup: Run or run/walk to location for Basic Circuit	5
		Daily Dozen	12
		Basic Circuit x 3: Perform each of the following exercises for 40 seconds each, with 20 seconds of rest in between. One time through the list of exercises equals one circuit. Do 3 circuits with minimal rest in between circuits: Push-ups, Steam Engines on Back, Squats, Ranger Crawls, Jump Rope or Jumping Jacks, Burpees, Russian Twists, Shuttle Run	25
		Home Stretch	10
Day 4	55–85	**Daily Dozen**	12
		Tempo Workout: Choose a cardio activity you enjoy, such as running, fast walking, cycling, or swimming. For your Tempo Workout, do the following: **Warm Up**—10 minutes at an easy pace (around 50% of your maximum effort).	30–60

WEEK 9	TOTAL MINUTES	EXERCISE AND INTENSITY	MINUTES PER ROUTINE
		Tempo—Speed up your pace so that you are closer to 70% to 80% of your maximum effort. *Duration: Beginners—10 minutes Intermediate—20 minutes Advanced—30 minutes*	
		Cool Down—10 minutes at an easy pace	
		Or Cross Train: Daily Dozen plus 2 minutes of cardio exercise between each routine (running, jumping rope, jumping jacks, fast walking, run/walk, or similar)	
		Home Stretch	10
DAY 5	50–55	**Circuit Training:**	
		Cardio Warmup: Run or run/walk to location for Basic Circuit	5
		Daily Dozen	12
		Basic Circuit x 3: Perform each of the following exercises for 40 seconds each, with 20 seconds of rest in between. One time through the list of exercises equals one circuit. Do 3 circuits with minimal rest in between circuits: Push-ups, Steam Engines on Back, Squats, Ranger Crawls, Jump Rope or Jumping Jacks, Burpees, Russian Twists, Shuttle Run	25
		Home Stretch	10
DAY 6	12	**Daily Dozen/Rest**	12
DAY 7	120	**Cornerstone Workout:** **The One Thousand**	120

the one thousand: inspiration

This is a workout that you can brag about when you go to the office on Monday morning. It's a significant amount of work, and as many times as we've done it, not one person has ever found it easy. There's a reason this workout comes in Week 9 and not Week 2. The One Thousand honors the concept of *thinking big*.

Some would say that the sheer amount of exercise involved in this workout is "too much." For some people, that would be true. However, keep in mind Challenge by Choice, along with the fact that you are now well-practiced on the fundamental and foundational movements and exercises.

The One Thousand could be seen as a "breakthrough workout"—a workout that helps you take a massive step forward in your fitness. You may find that when you get to the 600th repetition, you feel you've bitten off more than you can chew, but this is the very point of the One Thousand. You feel that you might not necessarily have what it takes to complete the exercise and so, in a very controlled way, you create an opportunity to dig deep into your reserves and find out what you're made of.

One thing is for sure: as you struggle through the last minutes of this workout, you will have put yourself, metaphorically speaking, into the shoes of a champion athlete when they've made their winning move. They've committed to the work involved, set their sights on the finish, and are now in the process of producing the best effort that they can muster. The next workout will seem considerably easier, simply because you've now reframed your entire concept of what the word "hard" really means.

WEEK 9: DAY BY DAY

DAY 1

You know what to do: your **Daily Dozen** followed by your moderate-intensity **endurance activity.** You have 45 to 180 minutes to play with—as always, use this as a Challenge by Choice moment and do what feels best to you.

DAY 2

Start your day with the **Daily Dozen,** and then enjoy some **restoration and relaxation.**

DAY 3

Time for your Basic Circuit workout. Set aside around 1 hour for this workout. **Run for 5 minutes** to a location for your circuit, perform your **Daily Dozen,** and then perform 3 rounds of the **Basic Circuit** (see the workout chart for the exercise list). Finish with your **Home Stretch.**

DAY 4

Another chance to practice Challenge by Choice: tackle your Tempo Workout or your outdoor Cross-Training Workout. Same guidelines as in previous weeks: you can do the same **Cross-Training Workout** you've done so far in this program, or perform half of your favorite Cornerstone Workout. If you choose a **Tempo Workout,** remember to warm up at moderate intensity for 10 minutes, and then push your pace with your desired cardio activity: 10 minutes for beginners, 20 for intermediate athletes, and 30 minutes for advanced athletes, going at around 70 percent to 80 percent of maximum effort. Finish with 10 minutes at an easy pace to cool down, and top it off with your **Home Stretch**.

DAY 5

Same as Day 3: the Basic Circuit workout. **Run for 5 minutes** to a location for your circuit, perform your **Daily Dozen,** and then perform three rounds of the **Basic Circuit** (see the workout chart for the exercise list). Finish with your **Home Stretch.**

DAY 6

Start your day with the **Daily Dozen**. For the rest of the day, enjoy a time of **restoration and relaxation.**

DAY 7

Time for the **One Thousand Cornerstone Workout.** Workout details follow.

THE ONE THOUSAND: THE CORNERSTONE WORKOUT

GEAR LIST
▪ Your usual kit: a sports watch, water, energy snack, small notebook and pen, first-aid kit, cell phone, and sun protection if necessary.
▪ Two rocks (about 5 pounds each) or resistance bands for bicep and shoulder exercises.
▪ Five cones or rocks to mark exercise stations (optional).

IDEAL TERRAIN
▪ Soft, grassy terrain for all exercises.
▪ A picnic bench or a set of stairs for Triceps Dips. (If none is available, you can perform this exercise on the ground.)

THE EXERCISES:
▪ For the Daily Dozen exercises, turn to page 67.
▪ For the Home Stretch exercises, turn to page 75.
▪ For all other exercises, turn to Appendix A, "Compendium of Exercises," page 223.

THE ONE THOUSAND: MINUTE BY MINUTE

 00:00 to 00:10
Run or run/walk to your warmup area. Today we'll jump right into it: perform 10 reps each of the following 10 exercises as your **calisthenic warmup.** This also counts as your first 100 reps in your One Thousand.
▪ Steam Engines
▪ Toe Touchers
▪ Twisters
▪ Side Benders
▪ Squats
▪ Lunges
▪ Crocodiles
▪ Scissors
▪ Push-ups
▪ Steam Engines on Back

00:10 to 00:25

Now, **run for about 5 minutes** to another grassy, soft area (or run out and back to the same area where you did your first 100 repetitions) for repetitions 101 to 200. Do 2 circuits of the following 5 exercises, 10 reps each time, for a total of 100 reps.

- Mountain Climbers
- Lunges
- Squats
- Side Lunges
- Squat Thrusters

00:25 to 00:35

Run for another 5 minutes, this time to an area that includes a picnic bench, steps, or a log for Triceps Dips, if available. The following **upper-body circuit**, 10 reps each exercise, takes you to 300 in your quest for the One Thousand.

- Push-ups
- Triceps Dips
- Push-ups variation: Wide Arm
- Triceps Dips
- Push-ups variation: Diamond
- Push-ups (normal)
- Triceps Dips
- Push-ups variation: Wide Arm
- Triceps Dips
- Push-ups variation: Diamond

00:35 to 00:55

Run for 10 minutes to another soft grassy surface, or head back toward the area you used earlier. The following **power circuit** (so named because it involves exercises that develop power and speed) gives you another 100 reps (10 reps each exercise):

- Burpees
- Mountain Climbers
- Lunges
- Squat Thrusters
- Triceps Dips
- Side Plank with Arm Twist—5 reps each side

- Push-ups—try the plyometric variety if you're so inclined
- Shuttle Run (20 yards)
- Power Jumps
- Scissor Jumps

🕐 **00:55 to 01:05**

Another circuit in the same location. Take a moment to rest between circuits before starting this **upper-body circuit.** Find two rocks or other heavy objects (around 5 pounds each) for your Military Presses and Biceps Curls—or carry a resistance band with you for those exercises. Do 2 full circuits of 10 reps for each exercise listed below and you'll be at 500 reps for the day, and counting.

- Arm Extenders
- Biceps Curls
- Military Presses
- Seagulls
- Arm Circles

🕐 **01:05 to 01:15**

Run for 5 minutes, up a hill or stairs if the terrain is available to you. At the top of the hill, **do 2 complete circuits** of 10 reps of each of the following exercises for your core circuit.

- Crocodiles
- Scissors
- Dolphins
- Steam Engines on Back
- Push-outs

🕐 **01:15 to 01:25**

Now, **run for another 5 minutes** to an area with a picnic bench for Triceps Dips. Do **2 circuits of the following exercises** for, you guessed it, 10 reps each. That brings you to 700 reps for the day.

- Push-ups
- Lunges
- Burpees variation: Projectile Burpees
- Power Hops
- Triceps Dips

01:25 to 01:35

Now it's your turn! **Run for 5 minutes,** and then pick **your 10 favorite exercises.** Do 10 reps of each exercise to get to 800 reps for the day.

01:35 to 01:45

Our last effort circuit of the day. **Run for another 5 minutes,** and then set up cones or rocks at **5 exercise "stations"** in a field, about 50 yards apart. Do the following 5 exercises, 10 reps each, twice around the cone stations, to get to 900 reps for the day.

- Triceps Dips
- Push-ups
- Steam Engines on Back
- Burpees
- Jumping Jacks

01:45 to 02:00

We're almost there! **Run for your final 5 minutes** of the workout to your **Home Stretch** location. Hold each stretch for 10 seconds (we'll count them as 10 reps each). That's a full One Thousand exercises for the day. When you're finished, top off your workout with your five full breaths of Final Breathing. That's it—you've completed the One Thousand! Well done.

- Upper Calf Stretch
- Lower Calves and Ankles
- Hamstrings
- Quadriceps
- Hip Flexors
- Thigh Adductors
- Back Stretch
- Stomach and Chest Stretch
- Triceps Stretch
- Shoulder Stretch

week 10 the triple ten high-intensity workout

Ten weeks in and we're going long for the third straight week, but in a new way. You'll do your usual week of conditioning, followed by a short, sweet, but 100 percent intense Cornerstone Workout. Pace yourself, remember your commitment to Challenge by Choice, and have a great time.

WEEK 10: FIRST NOTES

You'll continue your workout program with a week of solid conditioning before diving into the Triple Ten Cornerstone Workout. This workout takes many of the strengths, skills, and techniques that you have developed over the past 10 weeks and puts them to the test in a high-intensity workout. We suggest that you use weights for this workout. They can be as light as 2 pounds each for beginners; for someone in top shape, 10-pound dumbbells work well. Very few people will need heavier weights than 10 pounds to make this workout very effective. You can get inexpensive dumbbells at a local sporting goods store, or you can use water jugs with handles, or even rocks.

The Triple Ten is as much a fitness concept as it is a workout. The goal is to stay in motion, performing challenging movements, for 20 to 27 minutes consecutively. The primary physical benefit is that your muscle endurance will skyrocket, but you'll also receive the mental benefit of knowing you're getting stronger by the minute—this workout reaps massive benefits very quickly. You can do the Triple Ten in many different ways—we present no less than four different variations on the exercises below—but the reason behind the workout is to provide another type of high-quality workout that builds variety into your program.

One of the major advantages of the Triple Ten is that it can be done in a very small space, in a short amount of time—you'll be starting your cooldown by the time you reach the 55-minute mark of this Cornerstone

Workout. The exercises can be interchanged; you'll find your own circuits to use for this workout in the future. As long as you're doing 10 exercises, for 10 repetitions each, and repeating the entire circuit 10 times (10x10x10), you've got it.

the triple ten: inspiration

Ten weeks is a significant amount of time to train. You have built endurance, strength, and confidence. This week's workout, the Triple Ten, is one you can do anywhere, but why not choose a really inspiring location to push you through? You could do the workout alone, but this one works particularly well with a workout partner—being able to cheer on your partners while you're pushing yourself harder than you've ever worked in a Cornerstone Workout will create tons of positive energy, and a positive result can only follow from that.

WEEK 10: WORKOUT CHART

WEEK 10	TOTAL MINUTES	EXERCISE AND INTENSITY	MINUTES PER ROUTINE
Day 1	60–195	**Daily Dozen**	12
		Cardiovascular Endurance Moderate intensity (running, biking, hiking, swimming, fast walking, or a combination)	45–180
Day 2	12	**Daily Dozen/Rest**	12
Day 3	50–55	**Circuit Training:**	
		Cardio Warmup: Run or run/walk to location for Basic Circuit	5
		Daily Dozen	12
		Basic Circuit x 3: Perform each of the following exercises for 40 seconds each, with 20 seconds of rest in between. One time through the list of exercises equals one circuit. Do 3 circuits with minimal rest in between circuits: Push-ups, Steam Engines on Back, Squats, Ranger Crawls, Jump Rope or Jumping Jacks, Burpees, Russian Twists, Shuttle Run	25
		Home Stretch	10
Day 4	55–85	**Daily Dozen**	12
		Tempo Workout: Choose a cardio activity you enjoy, such as running, fast walking, cycling, or swimming. For your Tempo Workout, do the following: **Warm Up**—10 minutes at an easy pace (around 50% of your maximum effort).	30–60

WEEK 10	TOTAL MINUTES	EXERCISE AND INTENSITY	MINUTES PER ROUTINE
		Tempo—Speed up your pace so that you are closer to 70% to 80% of your maximum effort. *Duration: Beginners—10 minutes Intermediate—20 minutes Advanced—30 minutes*	
		Cool Down—10 minutes at an easy pace	
		Or Cross Train: Daily Dozen plus 2 minutes of cardio exercise between each routine (running, jumping rope, jumping jacks, fast walking, run/walk, or similar)	
		Home Stretch	10
DAY 5	50–55	**Circuit Training:**	
		Cardio Warmup: Run or run/walk to location for Basic Circuit	5
		Daily Dozen	12
		Basic Circuit x 3: Perform each of the following exercises for 40 seconds each, with 20 seconds of rest in between. One time through the list of exercises equals one circuit. Do 3 circuits with minimal rest in between circuits: Push-ups, Steam Engines on Back, Squats, Ranger Crawls, Jump Rope or Jumping Jacks, Burpees, Russian Twists, Shuttle Run	25
		Home Stretch	10
DAY 6	12	**Daily Dozen/Rest**	12
DAY 7	120	**Cornerstone Workout: Triple Ten High-Intensity Workout**	120

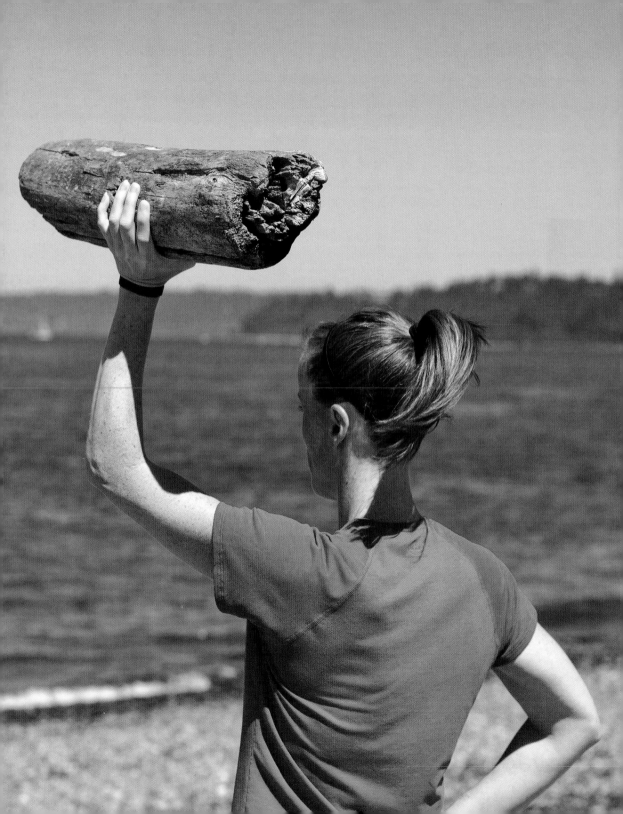

WEEK 10: DAY BY DAY

DAY 1
You know what to do: your **Daily Dozen** followed by your moderate-intensity **endurance activity** for 45 to 180 minutes.

DAY 2
Start your day with the **Daily Dozen**, and then enjoy **restoration and relaxation**.

DAY 3
Time for your Basic Circuit workout. Set aside around 1 hour for this workout. **Run for 5 minutes** to a location for your circuit, perform your **Daily Dozen,** and then perform 3 rounds of the **Basic Circuit** (see the workout chart for the exercise list). Finish with your **Home Stretch.**

DAY 4
Time for either a Tempo Workout or your outdoor Cross-Training Workout. As always, you have choices for your **Cross-Training Workout:** you can do the same workout you've done so far in this program, or for variety, take one of the Cornerstone Workouts you've done so far and simply cut it in half, so that you're working out for 1 hour or so. For a **Tempo Workout,** remember to warm up at moderate intensity for 10 minutes, and then push your pace with your desired cardio activity: 10 minutes for beginners, 20 for intermediate athletes, and 30 minutes for advanced athletes, going at around 70 percent to 80 percent of maximum effort. Finish with 10 minutes at an easy pace to cool down, and top it off with your **Home Stretch.**

DAY 5
Same as Day 3: the **Basic Circuit workout**. Run for 5 minutes to a location for your circuit, perform your **Daily Dozen,** and then perform 3 rounds of the **Basic Circuit** (see the workout chart above for the exercise list). Finish with your **Home Stretch.**

DAY 6
Start your day with the **Daily Dozen**. For the rest of the day, enjoy a time of **restoration and relaxation.**

DAY 7
Time for the **Triple Ten High-Intensity Cornerstone Workout.** Details follow.

THE TRIPLE TEN: THE CORNERSTONE WORKOUT

This workout is another variation on the circuit training you've done for the last 9 weeks. What makes this circuit different from the other circuits you've used so far in your training is that you will repeat the entire circuit 10 times. When you do the math, you'll see that this is quite similar to the One Thousand—with two major differences. One, each set of 10 exercises is the same. And two, we're asking you to take no rest in between each set of 10 exercises. This is a workout of constant movement that will require you to really pay attention to pacing yourself appropriately through the workout.

GEAR LIST
- Your usual kit: a sports watch, water, energy snack, small notebook and pen, first-aid kit, cell phone, and sun protection if necessary.
- A resistance band or a pair of weights (2 to 10 pounds, depending on your strength and fitness level). Alternatively, a pair of similarly sized rocks at your workout location works well.

IDEAL TERRAIN
- A flat, soft surface such as a grassy field.

THE EXERCISES:
- For the Daily Dozen exercises, turn to page 67.
- For the Home Stretch exercises, turn to page 75.
- For all other exercises, turn to Appendix A, "Compendium of Exercises," page 223.

THE TRIPLE TEN: MINUTE BY MINUTE

00:00 to 00:20
To get started, do your usual warmup: a **10-minute run or run/walk,** followed

by your **Daily Dozen**. For this workout in particular, take a few minutes to breathe, focus on your form and good core stability, and make sure to maintain a neutral spine throughout the movements. Paying close attention to the quality of your movement and maintaining good form will pay off for you in this workout.

🕐 **00:20 to 00:30**

Take another 10 minutes to **run or run/walk** to a destination with a flat, soft surface. When you reach your workout location, **relax** and visualize a great workout. The Triple Ten will ask a lot of you, so take time to gather your energy.

🕐 **00:30 to 00:55**

Next, you'll perform the **Triple Ten**—a set of 10 exercises of 10 repetitions each. This will likely take around 20 to 27 minutes to complete. The sidebar "Continuous High Intensity" on page 186 explains the Triple Ten and how to choose your circuit. If you find that you can do the entire Triple Ten in less than 20 minutes, increase the weight you use the next time around. If you find that it takes you longer than 27 minutes, decrease the weight next time. It's also perfectly fine to do this workout with no weight at all. You might want to try holding a light stick in each hand instead of weights the first time you perform this workout in order to simply get used to holding something in your hands.

🕐 **00:55 to 01:00**

Take 5 to 10 minutes for a **very light run or walk** to start your cooldown process. You can either come back to the same grassy area you used for your Triple Ten, or go back to your original location where you did your warmup and Daily Dozen.

🕐 **01:00 to 01:10**

Do your **Home Stretch**, paying particular attention to holding each stretch for a solid 10 to 20 seconds. You've just taxed your body to a very high degree, so make sure that you take the time to stretch yourself out and to fully cool down before heading out for the rest of your day. Congratulations—this was your toughest Cornerstone Workout yet.

continuous high intensity

Choose one of the ten circuits listed below for your **Triple Ten.** You will perform ten repetitions of each exercise. This type of workout is known as continuous high intensity. It requires maximum focus, energy, and no small amount of mental toughness. The rewards you'll get from dedicating yourself to this workout are impressive: increased muscle endurance, increased cardiovascular strength, and an increased awareness of how your body performs under pressure.

Depending on your own perceived level of fitness (beginner, intermediate, or advanced), select one of the circuits below. Note that some of the exercises will require light weights or resistance bands. If you're in a park without access to weights, look for a pair of similarly sized rocks to use for the strength moves. (Turn to Appendix A, "Compendium of Exercises," for detailed and illustrated instructions about how to perform each exercise. Take the time to learn each exercise thoroughly before you begin the Triple Ten circuit.)

	Beginner	Intermediate	Advanced (The Power Ten)
1	Three-quarter Squats	Three-quarter Squats	Burpees
2	Squat and Reach	Deadlifts	Mountain Climbers
3	Arm Extenders	Upright Rows	Push-ups
4	Lunges	Biceps Curls	Power Jumps
5	Jumping Jacks	Military Presses	Side Planks with Arm Twist (5 on each side)
6	Push-ups	Sumo Squats	Cleans
7	Side Benders	Squat Jumps	Squat Thrusters
8	Russian Twists	Cleans	Wide-Arm Push-ups
9	Steam Engines	Squat Thrusters	Super Burpees
10	Plank (hold for 30 seconds)	Push-ups	Diamond Push-ups

If you're ready to make this circuit more difficult, you can increase the amount of weight you use for the exercises (e.g., around 10 pounds in each hand for the intermediate circuit). When you're ready for something even harder than the advanced circuit, you can perform the following advanced circuit with added weight:

Advanced Triple Ten Circuit with Weight

1	Squats
2	Deadlifts
3	Upright Rows
4	Biceps Curls
5	Military Presses
6	Squat Thrusters
7	Push-ups
8	Russian Twists
9	Steam Engines on Back
10	Squat Jumps (holding weights)

The goal is to perform each of the ten sets of the Triple Ten at the same pace. The easiest way to find a good pace when you're getting started is to do the first few runs through the exercise circuit at a pace that feels slower than you think you can do it. That will help you to keep from burning out in the middle. That said, if you do reach a point during the workout where you're extremely fatigued, simply take a minute or two to recover before moving forward.

This is one of the only Cornerstone Workouts presented in this book in which you can use weights for the exercises. If you have dumbbells, you can place them on the ground and hold them during your Push-ups and Squat Thrusters, and hold them in your hands for all other exercises. (Note that only intermediate or advanced athletes should hold weights in their hands when doing a jumping movement such as a Squat Jump.) As with all other Cornerstone Workouts, this class is all about Challenge by Choice. Test out what it feels like to hold weights and perform a Squat Jump before jumping into this workout.

week 11 put it to the test, part 2

Another week of conditioning will be followed by your second fitness test day in your twelve-week program. You're about to discover just how much fitter you are since you've been working out with adventX. Put on your favorite workout gear and get ready to impress.

WEEK 11: FIRST NOTES

The name of this workout week says it all—during this week's Cornerstone Workout, you'll quantify just how fit you've become in the last ten weeks. Remember that you are not just physically fitter, you're also mentally fitter. As you prepare to take your fitness tests, spend time visualizing what it feels like for an elite athlete to step into the arena at a major sports event. Of course there will be some nervousness—who wouldn't feel a little nervous in such a situation? You're likely to feel some excitement, anticipation, and the sense of your pulse racing. The antidote to nervousness is deep breathing, so take some full, deep breaths as you anticipate your fitness tests.

And as you do this, enjoy the moment. All athletes develop precompetition routines. Some use mantras, some a particular song, some funny thoughts, and some prayer. All of these mental strategies can calm you down before a big effort. If your mind comes up blank, think of where you started from and where you are now. Visualize the people in your life who are proud of your accomplishments (including yourself, of course).

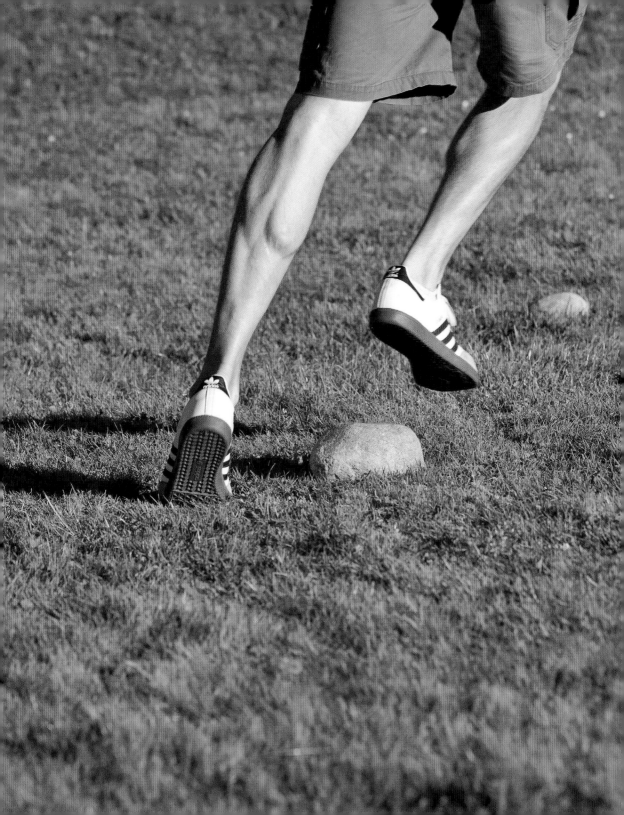

WEEK 11: WORKOUT CHART

WEEK 11	TOTAL MINUTES	EXERCISE AND INTENSITY	MINUTES PER ROUTINE
Day 1	60–195	**Daily Dozen**	12
		Cardiovascular Endurance Moderate intensity (running, biking, hiking, swimming, fast walking, or a combination)	45–180
Day 2	12	**Daily Dozen/Rest**	12
Day 3	50–55	**Circuit Training:**	
		Cardio Warmup: Run or run/walk to location for Basic Circuit	5
		Daily Dozen	12
		Basic Circuit x 3: Perform each of the following exercises for 40 seconds each, with 20 seconds of rest in between. One time through the list of exercises equals one circuit. Do 3 circuits with minimal rest in between circuits: Push-ups, Steam Engines on Back, Squats, Ranger Crawls, Jump Rope or Jumping Jacks, Burpees, Russian Twists, Shuttle Run	25
		Home Stretch	10
Day 4	55–85	**Daily Dozen**	12
		Tempo Workout: Choose a cardio activity you enjoy, such as running, fast walking, cycling, or swimming. For your Tempo Workout, do the following: **Warm Up**—10 minutes at an easy pace (around 50% of your maximum effort).	30–60

WEEK 11	TOTAL MINUTES	EXERCISE AND INTENSITY	MINUTES PER ROUTINE
		Tempo—Speed up your pace so that you are closer to 70% to 80% of your maximum effort. *Duration: Beginners—10 minutes Intermediate—20 minutes Advanced—30 minutes*	
		Cool Down—10 minutes at an easy pace	
		Or Cross Train: Daily Dozen plus 2 minutes of cardio exercise between each routine (running, jumping rope, jumping jacks, fast walking, run/walk, or similar)	
		Home Stretch	10
DAY 5	50–55	**Circuit Training:**	
		Cardio Warmup: Run or run/walk to location for Basic Circuit	5
		Daily Dozen	12
		Basic Circuit x 3: Perform each of the following exercises for 40 seconds each, with 20 seconds of rest in between. One time through the list of exercises equals one circuit. Do 3 circuits with minimal rest in between circuits: Push-ups, Steam Engines on Back, Squats, Ranger Crawls, Jump Rope or Jumping Jacks, Burpees, Russian Twists, Shuttle Run	25
		Home Stretch	10
DAY 6	12	**Daily Dozen/Rest**	12
DAY 7	120	**Cornerstone Workout: Put It to the Test**	120

WEEK 11: DAY BY DAY

DAY 1

You know what to do: your **Daily Dozen**, followed by your moderate-intensity **cardiovascular endurance activity** for 45 to 180 minutes.

DAY 2

Start your day with the **Daily Dozen**, and then enjoy a day of **restoration and relaxation.**

DAY 3

Time for your Basic Circuit workout. Set aside around 1 hour for this workout. **Run for 5 minutes** to a location for your circuit, perform your **Daily Dozen,** and then perform 3 rounds of the **Basic Circuit** (see the workout chart for the exercise list). Finish with your **Home Stretch.**

DAY 4

Time for either a Tempo Workout or your outdoor Cross-Training Workout. You have choices for your **Cross-Training Workout:** you can do the same workout you've done so far in this program, or for variety, take one of the Cornerstone Workouts you've done so far and simply cut it in half, so that you're working out for 1 hour or so. Remember your **Tempo Workout** guidelines: warm up at moderate intensity for 10 minutes, and then push your pace with your desired cardio activity: 10 minutes for beginners, 20 for intermediate athletes, and 30 minutes for advanced athletes, going at around 70 percent to 80 percent of maximum effort. Finish with 10 minutes at an easy pace to cool down, and top it off with your **Home Stretch.**

DAY 5

Same as Day 3: **Run for 5 minutes** to a location for your circuit, perform your **Daily Dozen,** and then perform 3 rounds of the **Basic Circuit** (see the workout chart for the exercise list). Finish with your **Home Stretch.**

DAY 6:

Start your day with the **Daily Dozen**. For the rest of the day, enjoy a time of **restoration and relaxation.**

DAY 7

Ready for a great challenge? It's time for your **Put It to the Test, Part 2 Cornerstone Workout.** Details below.

PUT IT TO THE TEST, PART 2: THE CORNERSTONE WORKOUT

GEAR LIST

- Your usual kit: a sports watch, water, energy snack, small notebook and pen, first-aid kit, cell phone, and sun protection if necessary.
- Cones (if available); otherwise, a rock or water bottle will do.

IDEAL TERRAIN

- Your favorite timed-run course.
- A flat, grassy, soft surface such as an athletic field.

THE EXERCISES:

- For the Daily Dozen exercises, turn to page 67.
- For the Home Stretch exercises, turn to page 75.
- For all other exercises, turn to Appendix A, "Compendium of Exercises," page 223.

PUT IT TO THE TEST, PART 2: MINUTE BY MINUTE

🕐 **00:00 to 00:20**
Run or run/walk for 10 minutes, then do your **Daily Dozen.** Have fun and feel the benefit of all the training you've done as you warm up your body.

🕐 **00:20 to 00:30**
Head for the location of your **timed run**—preferably the same timed run you used in Week 4. As you move toward the course, do some warmup running drills: Butt Kicks, High Knees, Side to Side Strides, Backwards Running, and Skipping.

00:30 to 00:32

When you've reached your timed-run location, take two full minutes to **be still and get ready for your run**.

00:32 to 00:40 (approximately)

When you're centered and focused and have taken complete ownership of your thoughts, you're ready for your **timed run**. Start your watch and go! Remember to break the run into segments—focus on each quarter of the run, or visualize running 100 yards 16 times, rather than a whole mile. At the half-way point, check in with yourself. Keep your head up with hips and shoulders squared to the direction you're running, with hands and arms relaxed. Before you know it, you'll have just 30 to 40 seconds left in your run. Relax and let yourself float to the finish line on momentum.

00:40 to 00:50

Take time to **recover** after this run. Record your time, and take a full rest period of at least 5 minutes. Drink water, and perhaps a few sips of a sports drink. Once you're ready, walk or run to a grassy, soft spot where you'll do the other 4 exercises in the fitness test.

00:50 to 01:10

The remainder of the fitness test is the same exact thing you did in Week 4: **4 exercises, each done for 2 minutes**, with a 4-minute break in between each exercise. The exercises are Push-ups, Burpees, Steam Engines on Back, and the 20-yard Shuttle Run.

Remember to count the number of full repetitions of each exercise that you're able to do in 2 minutes. Also, keep in mind that these exercises can be challenging, even at an advanced state of fitness. You'll want to go fast and hard, but pace yourself—if you begin too quickly, your body could shut down before you finish your 2 minutes. It's pace, not distance, that will make or break this workout.

01:10 to 01:15

You've just finished not simply an incredible workout, but a significant effort in your fitness journey. **Walk** to your Home Stretch location. You've done enough hard work for today.

01:15 to 01:25

Home Stretch. And you're done—relax for the rest of the day and enjoy your accomplishment.

put it to the test, part 2: inspiration

What we said in Week 4 when you did your first fitness test applies to this week as well: it's all about quantifying your progress, a very helpful tool especially for athletes who tend to be too hard on themselves.

Do you ever feel like you're tough on yourself because you're not performing "strong enough" or "fast enough"? Consider moving away from quantifying your progress based on incomplete perceptions. The fitness test gives you measurable results—*real* results that you can refer back to again and again as you continue your fitness adventure throughout your life. You might choose to keep track of year-by-year fitness test results, or lifetime personal bests, or personal bests for each birthday or decade. I've seen time and time again that athletes who focus on specific, measurable achievements will easily achieve more than their counterparts who don't set these kinds of strong goals. Have a great time out there with this Cornerstone Workout, and remember to record your marks.

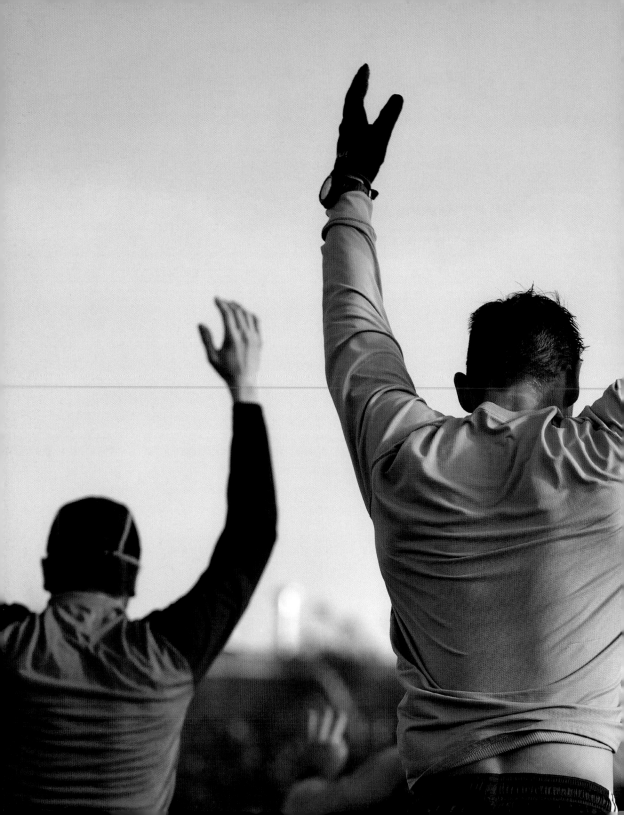

week 12 peak performance

The final workout week of the season—a chance to revisit some favorite moments from the preceding weeks, reach peak performance, and set goals for the next season.

WEEK 12: FIRST NOTES

You've reached your twelfth week of working out consistently, and you're ready to celebrate. The overall theme of the Peak Performance week is one of congratulations, reflection, and celebration.

WEEK 12: WORKOUT CHART

WEEK 12	TOTAL MINUTES	EXERCISE AND INTENSITY	MINUTES PER ROUTINE
Day 1	60–195	**Daily Dozen**	12
		Cardiovascular Endurance Moderate intensity (running, biking, hiking, swimming, fast walking, or a combination)	45–180
Day 2	12	**Daily Dozen/Rest**	12
Day 3	50–55	**Circuit Training:**	
		Cardio Warmup: Run or run/walk to location for Basic Circuit	5
		Daily Dozen	12
		Basic Circuit x 3: Perform each of the following exercises for 40 seconds each, with 20 seconds of rest in between. One time through the list of exercises equals one circuit. Do 3 circuits with minimal rest in between circuits: Push-ups, Steam Engines on Back, Squats, Ranger Crawls, Jump Rope or Jumping Jacks, Burpees, Russian Twists, Shuttle Run	25
		Home Stretch	10
Day 4	55–85	**Daily Dozen**	12
		Tempo Workout: Choose a cardio activity you enjoy, such as running, fast walking, cycling, or swimming. For your Tempo Workout, do the following: **Warm Up**—10 minutes at an easy pace (around 50% of your maximum effort).	30–60

WEEK 12	TOTAL MINUTES	EXERCISE AND INTENSITY	MINUTES PER ROUTINE

Tempo—Speed up your pace so that you are closer to 70% to 80% of your maximum effort.
Duration:
Beginners—10 minutes
Intermediate—20 minutes
Advanced—30 minutes

Cool Down—10 minutes at an easy pace

Or Cross Train: Daily Dozen plus 2 minutes of cardio exercise between each routine (running, jumping rope, jumping jacks, fast walking, run/walk, or similar)

		Home Stretch	10

DAY 5	50–55	**Circuit Training:**	
		Cardio Warmup: Run or run/walk to location for Basic Circuit	5
		Daily Dozen	12
		Basic Circuit x 3: Perform each of the following exercises for 40 seconds each, with 20 seconds of rest in between. One time through the list of exercises equals one circuit. Do 3 circuits with minimal rest in between circuits: Push-ups, Steam Engines on Back, Squats, Ranger Crawls, Jump Rope or Jumping Jacks, Burpees, Russian Twists, Shuttle Run	25
		Home Stretch	10
DAY 6	12	**Daily Dozen/Rest**	12
DAY 7	120	**Cornerstone Workout: Peak Performance**	120

WEEK 12: DAY BY DAY

DAY 1
It's the last cardiovascular endurance workout of the season: your **Daily Dozen** followed by your moderate-intensity **endurance activity** for 45 to 180 minutes.

DAY 2
Start with the **Daily Dozen,** and then enjoy a day of **restoration and relaxation.**

DAY 3
Time for your Basic Circuit workout. Set aside around 1 hour for this workout. **Run for 5 minutes** to a location for your circuit, perform your **Daily Dozen,** and then perform 3 rounds of the **Basic Circuit** (see the workout chart for the exercise list). Finish with your **Home Stretch.**

DAY 4
Choose a Tempo Workout or your outdoor Cross-Training Workout—try the one you've done least this season for today's effort. As always, for your **Cross-Training Workout,** you can do the same workout you've done so far in this program, or do half of your favorite Cornerstone Workout. For a **Tempo Workout,** warm up at moderate intensity for 10 minutes, and then push your pace with your desired cardio activity: 10 minutes for beginners, 20 for intermediate athletes, and 30 minutes for advanced athletes, going at around 70 percent to 80 percent of maximum effort. Finish with 10 minutes at an easy pace to cool down, and top it off with your **Home Stretch.**

DAY 5
Same as Day 3: **Run for 5 minutes** to a location for your circuit, perform your **Daily Dozen,** and then perform 3 rounds of the **Basic Circuit** (see the workout chart for the exercise list). Finish with your **Home Stretch.**

DAY 6
Start your day with the **Daily Dozen**. For the rest of the day, enjoy a time of **restoration and relaxation.**

DAY 7

Time for the **Peak Performance Cornerstone Workout,** the last one of the season. Details below.

PEAK PERFORMANCE: THE CORNERSTONE WORKOUT

GEAR LIST

▪ Your usual kit: a sports watch, water, energy snack, small notebook and pen, first-aid kit, cell phone, and sun protection if necessary.

IDEAL TERRAIN

▪ Choose your favorite workout area—a place that invigorates you. Feel free to adapt the Cornerstone Workout to this area if you would like, so that you're really ready to enjoy this last major workout of the season. And remember to take some time to smell the roses, as they say (or the pine cones, the grass, the air by the seashore, or whatever natural phenomena live in your neck of the woods).

THE EXERCISES:

▪ For the Daily Dozen exercises, turn to page 67.
▪ For the Home Stretch exercises, turn to page 75.
▪ For all other exercises, turn to Appendix A, "Compendium of Exercises," page 223.

PEAK PERFORMANCE: MINUTE BY MINUTE

 00:00 to 00:20
Do your usual workout—a **10-minute run or run/walk** followed by your **Daily Dozen**. Make this the best Daily Dozen you've ever done.

00:20 to 00:25
Run 5 minutes to find your first workout station. Today's workout will be made up of 10 segments, including the warmup/Daily Dozen and Home Stretch, so this is your second exercise segment of the day, and it will be a balance segment.

00:25 to 00:35
Perform **the following exercises** for 10 repetitions each, except where noted:

- Vector Toe Touches
- Single-Leg Side-to-Side Hops
- Thirsty Bird
- Supermans
- Standing on one leg, eyes closed—try this for one minute on each leg

 00:35 to 00:40
Next, **run for 2 minutes**, then perform 10 repetitions of each exercise in the following circuit:

- Push-ups
- Triceps Dips
- Push-ups
- Triceps Dips
- Push-ups

 00:40 to 00:45
Run 2 more minutes, then do the following **core circuit** (10 repetitions each exercise):

- Crocodiles
- Scissors
- Steam Engines on Back
- Dolphins
- Push-outs

 00:45 to 00:50
Run for 2 more minutes, then do the following quick **power circuit:**

- Mountain Climbers
- Power Jumps
- Push-ups
- Burpees
- Squat Thrusters

 00:50 to 00:55
Run for 2 more minutes, then repeat the **Push-up/Triceps Dip circuit** you

did at 00:35 (3 sets of Push-ups, with 2 sets of Triceps Dips interspersed between the sets of Push-ups, for 10 repetitions each exercise).

00:55 to 01:05
Break up the rhythm a bit. **Run lightly** for about 1 mile or 10 minutes.

01:05 to 01:10
Perform the following **core muscle circuit:**
- Russian Twists
- Push-outs
- Steam Engines
- Dolphins
- Side Plank with Arm Twist

peak performance: inspiration

This week's Cornerstone Workout is designed to do something very special: enable and empower you for future success. You've worked incredibly hard during this program. You've had the courage and commitment to begin, and the discipline to stick with it. You may have struggled, and you may have even wanted to quit. You've likely not done everything to your idea of perfection, but that's the point: there is no perfect in fitness. You have succeeded not by doing everything "right," but by doing the next right thing over and over again. You've experienced the success that comes through moderation and consistency. You've seen the level to which your body will adapt to new challenges, no matter what your age, shape, size, or fitness level. You've breathed in some fresh air, you've (hopefully) seen some sun, and perhaps you've felt some rain on your face. And we hope you've also surrounded yourself with some beautiful scenery and wildlife. You'll do this workout at a moderate and consistent pace that leaves you feeling invigorated. You can do this workout as hard as you like, but you don't have to do it as hard as you're capable of doing it, unless that's what your body craves.

01:10 to 01:15
Walk for 5 minutes to get your heart rate back down after a great effort.

01:15 to 01:25
The next segment will be a **combination sprint/power circuit**—you'll do 10 repetitions of each exercise, and after each exercise, you'll sprint for about 50 yards, then immediately perform the next exercise in the circuit.

- Power Hops
- Sprint 50 yards
- Lunges
- Sprint 50 yards
- Squat Thrusters
- Sprint 50 yards
- Side Lunges
- Sprint 50 yards
- Sumo Squats
- Sprint 50 yards

01:25 to 01:32
Next, run for 3 minutes and then **repeat the core superset** (Crocodiles, Scissors, Steam Engines on Back, Dolphins, and Push-outs), 10 reps for each.

01:32 to 01:35
There are only 2 exercise segments left in the class, and the next one is your choice. **Run for 2 minutes,** and then **choose your 5 favorite exercises** and perform 10 repetitions of each one.

01:35 to 01:45
Finally, **run lightly for 10 minutes** toward your Home Stretch location, paying attention to your natural surroundings once again. Admire the landscape, the weather, and the wildlife. Celebrate 12 weeks of outdoor workouts with this run, saying goodbye (just for a short time) to your favorite exercise landscapes. Finish your run at a grassy field where you can do your final Home Stretch of the season.

01:45 to 01:55
Home Stretch—and you're done!

final thoughts on the season

You've just completed twelve weeks of outdoor workouts. Take the next week to rest as completely as you wish. Perhaps you will feel an urge to take some vigorous walks, or even a light run. Keep up with your Daily Dozen, if that's something you want to do. What you're looking for now is a solid period of transition before you begin the next season. A change in seasons, especially in an area with very pronounced differences in weather and amount of light between the seasons, offers a profound opportunity for you to retool your goals and move forward, building on what you've accomplished in the last twelve weeks. As we look ahead, we'll talk more about setting new goals, looking ahead to the next season, and also how to tackle the inevitable challenges and setbacks that every athlete experiences in cycles of training, improvement, and accomplishment. You've reached the end of your first twelve weeks, but in fact, you've only just begun your journey to a lifetime of outdoor fitness.

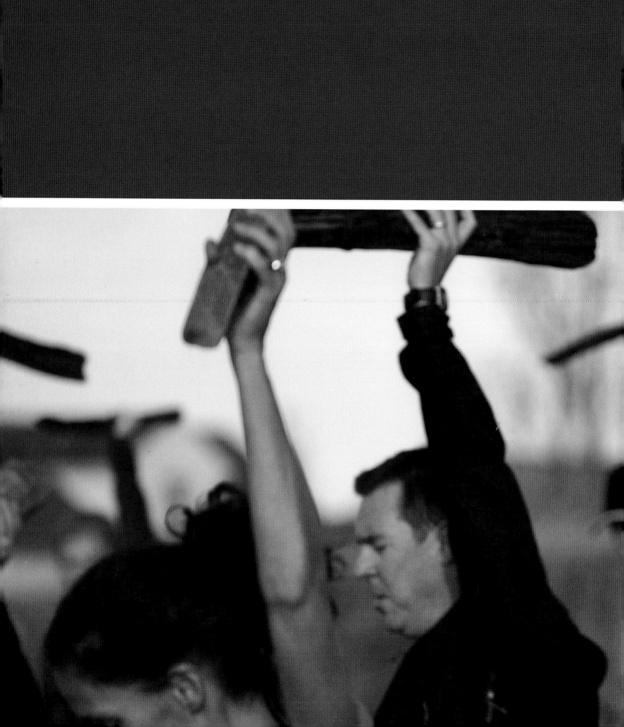

keep going

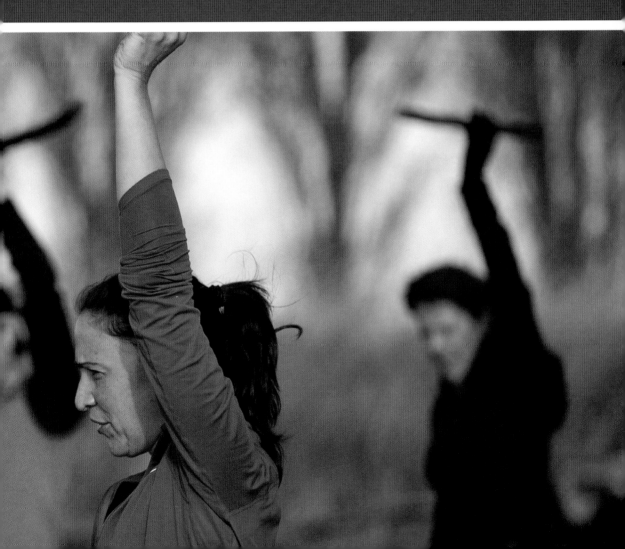

the next season

You've just worked out for an entire season in the outdoors. That's a tremendous accomplishment. According to the American College of Sports Medicine, less than 10 percent of people who begin a fitness program will still be following that program ninety days later. Congratulations—you're in a select group.

What next? You can look at the year as a series of **training phases**, much the same way we started by looking at a twelve-week period as a series of training phases. This will help you to visualize specific goals and tailor your training to each season, or phase, of your training. The program I describe below is an example, created for an athlete who wishes to peak for a multiday hike in late summer and a running race in early fall.

- Winter (January through March)—**Adapting.** This season will be used to get used to the training program.
- Spring (April through June)—**Building.** Athletes shift focus to build more aerobic endurance through longer Cardiovascular Endurance Workouts and more hill-based training in Cross-Training and Cornerstone Workouts.
- Summer (July through September)—**Peaking.** Athletes bring their training to a peak by working hard for the first half of the season, then gradually tapering training to about 50 percent to 60 percent of what it was during the hardest part of the season in order to rest for peak events: a multiday hike in late August or a running race in late September.
- Fall (October through December)—**Transitioning.** The late fall and early winter will be a time to dial back on hard training, allow the body to rest, and to do easier workouts at a lower intensity before setting new goals and beginning a new year of training.

As you can see from this example, phase-based training works both within a season and within a training year to give you a natural structure to plan out your workouts, goals, and **milestones**: the achievements along the way to a larger goal that demonstrate that your preparation is on target.

SETTING NEW GOALS

Consider two interrelated questions: what have you achieved in the last twelve weeks, and what would you like to do next? You have completed one massive improvement cycle. You've not only mastered the tasks of doing a great workout, but you've also planned, built and executed a successful twelve-week exercise program.

To more formally track your achievements, take a few minutes to redo the **adventX On-Target Questionnaire** (Appendix C) you completed before you began the program. Use your answers to compare yourself with where you were twelve weeks ago. Especially note the following:

- Areas where you felt significantly lacking twelve weeks ago but now feel competent (such as speed).
- Areas where you were already strong and now you feel stronger (such as flexibility).
- Areas that were lacking to begin with that still feel lacking (such as upper body strength).
- Areas that felt strong to begin with but that may now feel as though you've slipped backwards (such as balance).

From there, **look at the responses to your goal-setting questions** compared with your initial responses twelve weeks ago. Once you've looked at your goal-setting answers from the questionnaire, **pick one goal as your primary objective for the next three months.** According to many leading personal development experts, the chances of us reaching our goals are significantly higher when we write them down and communicate them than when we just hold them in our minds. If you're having trouble figuring out a primary goal, you may want to consult with a coach or a sports psychologist to discover what you want to achieve. Is it an event that you want to participate in? A race you'd like to run faster? Would you like to join new friends in an outdoor activity or join a club? Your goal will be as unique as you are. Then look at the list of the nine physiological strengths from the questionnaire and ask yourself which of those strengths will make the most difference to you in achieving your next goal.

After you've selected a primary goal, **set a secondary objective.** I've seen great success among adventX team members who create a primary objective and back it up with a secondary objective, and focus on achieving these goals in the space of a twelve-week workout cycle.

There is one more step to take in order to plan your next twelve-week program. Consider where you started and where you are now from a different angle. Which of these categories most closely represents you? Are you:

- A person who was not exercising regularly at all before beginning this program?
- A person who came to the program for general conditioning for a favorite sport or activity?
- A person who came to the program with a specific goal, achieved it, and is now ready to set a much more ambitious goal?

the power of goal-setting

I am always amazed at how different things can look in such a short period of time when you're striving for a goal. A tangible example of this is mountaineering. When I've climbed to around 14,000 feet on a 20,000-foot mountain and looked down over the clouds and valleys, I think the view couldn't be more spectacular. But then I look down two days later from 18,000 feet, and it's not only as beautiful but immeasurably *more* spectacular. Everything I thought was amazing and as good as it was ever going to get had just been eclipsed by something even more amazing. When you absorb the fact that our minds really are limited by what we see and have seen, and that as a result it's very difficult to imagine what could be in the future, you'll start to truly harness the power of goal-setting.

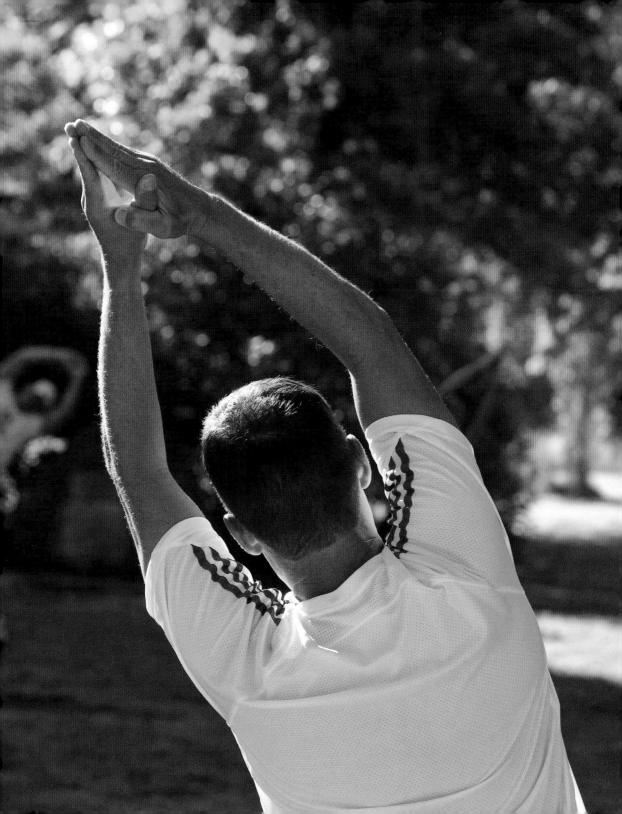

If you weren't exercising regularly before beginning the program, you'll want to take one week off for restoration and relaxation, and **repeat the entire twelve-week program,** keeping in mind your new goals. This next season will be entirely different, in no small part because the season has changed, and the terrain and weather will be different. Apply equal energy to all aspects of the program. Think about your goals, but don't worry too much about emphasizing one strength over another. Remember that it's the act of getting out there and working out that will result in success.

If you're the second type listed above, you had a good sense of what you were going to get in this program, and you received it. For instance, you may have picked up this book so that you could be in better shape for skiing, hiking, cycling, or triathlon training. I hope that you can immediately feel the benefits of this program for your sport. For your second twelve-week cycle, **shift into your main training for your sport or activity.** You can either revisit the twelve-week program this time next year when you want to improve your general conditioning, or you can take elements of the program that work for you and incorporate those into your training week during your sport's main season. You can also do your Daily Dozen every day, of course. If you love the idea of a weekly Cornerstone Workout in addition to training for your main sport, you can pick and choose the workouts you'd like to follow, or shorten the Cornerstone Workout by doing fewer repetitions of exercises, or just the first half of the workout. One more variation would be to continue with another twelve-week cycle, but do fewer workouts each week instead of the full program, so as to fit in your other sports.

If you're the third type of person, great! In that case, you'll want to **repeat the twelve-week program, but with an entirely different goal than you set the first time around.** You'll work a bit harder, move a little faster, but still have the structure that comes from following the prescribed program. If you feel particularly strong, you can **replace easier exercises with harder ones.** See Appendix B on sport-specific circuits for ideas for how to personalize your own program, and spend time with the Compendium of Exercises (Appendix A) as well, to look for more challenging movements to incorporate.

challenges, setbacks, and opportunities

The entire purpose of the adventX outdoor workout program is to enhance your life. But life throws us all kinds of curve balls that can keep us from attaining our goals if we give them the power to do so. How do you stay focused when your child has kept you up the last three nights with a cold and your boss is breathing down your neck?

In this book, we strive to give you equal parts explanation and inspiration to help you get into the outdoors for the benefit of your entire life. But there's a third ingredient to any successful fitness program: a reality check. In a perfect world, you can carve out two hours every Saturday for your Cornerstone Workouts and always have access to nutritious food at every turn. But that's not the world that I live in, and I bet you don't, either. I've seen athletes overcome what could seem to be stunning challenges, including life-changing illness and injuries. We hope that some of the material that follows helps you overcome life's stumbling blocks and stay focused on your overall fitness and health goals.

How do we adapt, improvise, and move forward with our fitness goals, even when we incur setbacks? Part of what we're going to do in this chapter is to provide you with practical tools that you can employ anytime to ensure that you achieve success and that you do everything you can to stay on an upward spiral.

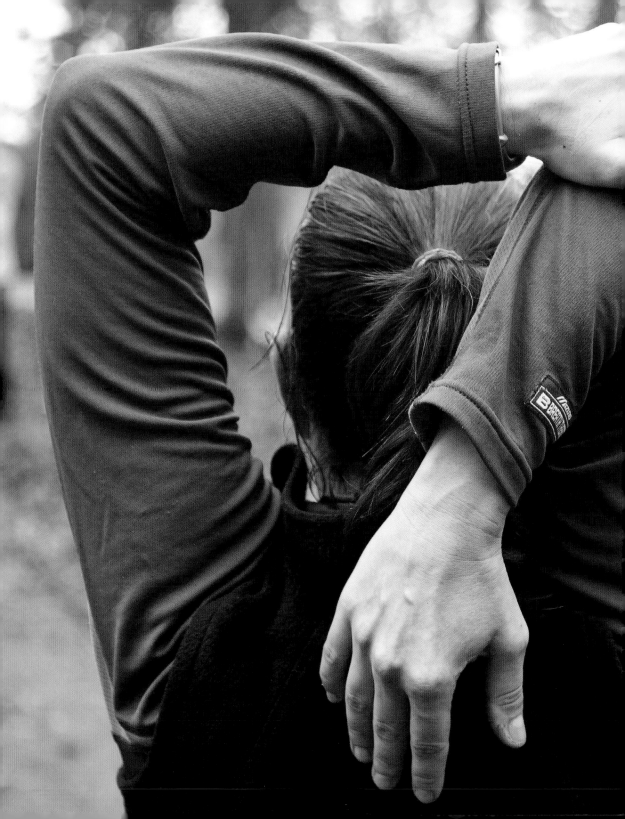

BUILDING FLEXIBILITY INTO YOUR PROGRAM: THE 80 PERCENT RULE

Perhaps the most important tool of all is to build flexibility into your program. I use the "80 percent rule" when writing out a training plan for a new client: if that athlete were to complete 80 percent of this training program, it's likely that he or she would gain exactly the results they desired. That brings up an obvious question: why not prescribe less exercise in the first place? We specifically designed the program with 20 percent leeway for exactly these types of challenges. It's unrealistic to adopt a training program where you have to achieve 100 percent of everything every day. This adds immense pressure to succeed in a way most people would find very difficult, and would not honor the fact that you're human, nor would it be a very sensible plan. Consider the entire twelve-week program in its entirety—if you miss two workouts in a given week because of extenuating life circumstances, you're well within your 20 percent leeway.

CHALLENGES: WHEN TRAINING JUST ISN'T GOING YOUR WAY

Many athletes feel as though they are to blame when they can't get enthused about working out. There are all kinds of reasons why your body might be telling you to slow down or even stop for a while: burnout, exhaustion, injuries, or just the natural changes that occur with the seasons. I often notice our athletes becoming just a step slower as the seasons change from summer to fall and the darkness of the mornings descends on us. We've outlined a few of the most common reasons you might feel challenged to complete your twelve-week program, and strategies for overcoming those challenges.

SETBACKS: WHEN LIFE GETS IN THE WAY OF TRAINING

Sometimes life hands us a bigger challenge than just burnout, sluggishness, or a bad race. Life can deal out some tremendously difficult cards sometimes—such as the end of a relationship, a death in your family or circle of

challenge: lack of workout enthusiasm

You're feeling sluggish with your training—perhaps you've had a bad day, or a bad week, or even a bad month, where your enthusiasm for working out wanes.

Potential Solutions: Are you exercising regularly, even if you start out feeling sluggish? Are you following a good nutrition program? Are you well hydrated? Are you getting enough sleep (seven to eight hours per night)? Are you paying attention to your stress level, perhaps planning in time for relaxation and restoration, perhaps even a brief nap if necessary? Are you surrounding yourself with a positive environment that supports your goals?

Ask yourself whether you're staying away from things that would be an impediment to those goals, like smoking, drinking to excess, or eating junk foods.

Usually when a person has this type of problem, there's a factor in the person's lifestyle or self-care program that is lacking. If you feel sluggish, go through the list above, perhaps taking some notes on your first impressions of each health aspect listed (exercise, nutrition, hydration, sleep, stress, and a positive environment). Do you feel like you are practicing good self-care? If you've taken a look at the list and you're still not sure what's causing your sluggishness, check it out with your doctor—many people have thyroid or other health issues that can be identified and addressed.

Next, think about your goals. Simply put, have you set appropriate goals? Do they motivate you? Is this a good time to look at it? What spurred the initial goal? You may have set a goal that's too ambitious (for example, a specific time for a difficult race) and you're overtraining. Look again at your goals and ask yourself if you can ramp down a bit to give yourself the leeway we talked about earlier. Sometimes giving yourself permission to scale back—Challenge by Choice, remember?—is all it takes to get your energy back.

challenge: burnout

After you've reached a big goal, it's normal for your body to effectively say "no more." History provides us with endless stories of adventurers and athletes of all levels who feel burned out after they've accomplished a significant goal. Our belief is that training outdoors enables us to better adapt to fluctuating energy and moods because we see the change in seasons first hand, as the natural world cycles from summer to fall to winter to spring.

Potential Solutions: Plan for the fact that after a big event, you might have a week or two when you want to take time off. A lot of professional athletes will go on vacation after a big event, just to change their environment. If you can't do that, do something completely different for a few weeks. If you spent Sundays doing long runs, for example, you can plan for an hour-long walk and nothing more on Sundays for the next few weeks.

Another thing that can be useful is to focus on the quality of the experience you've had. You've just spent weeks and months striving for a huge goal. Now, you can think about another goal—perhaps working on your upper-body strength, learning how to do pull-ups, going to a new exercise class you haven't done before, or taking up a new activity like yoga or kickboxing. Honor the fact that what felt good about the buildup to your event could be related to the purposefulness and intention that went along with the training. That passion will not exist at the same level after the event. Find purpose in your training, whether it be in exercise or perhaps even in another, unrelated activity—a hobby or work project, for example.

challenge: a bad race

However you define the experience, a bad race (or a mountain climb where you didn't reach the summit, or a triathlon you had to drop out of because of cramping) is a disappointment, no question.

Solution: Reframing. In situations like this, we ask athletes to reframe the experience to see it from a different perspective. One athlete recently ran her first marathon in nine years. She had been running well and had even set a personal best at a half-marathon two weeks before the big race. Success seemed assured, until mile nine, when her legs seized up with cramps. She considered dropping out but very much wanted to finish, so she walked as much as she needed to and finished, but nowhere near her goal time. Understandably, she was quite disappointed with her performance.

That's where reframing came into play. I asked her to see the race from the perspective of the spectators. Just running a marathon is nothing to sneeze at—and in fact only a tiny percentage of the population ever finishes a marathon at all. I reminded her that she was a lot further along than all the people who never started the race in the first place. Most people do not exercise. Just by starting, we're already in the top ten percent. So if you're in the middle of your exercise group, you're not halfway down the pile—you're halfway down a pile made up of the top ten percent of your peers. Reframing her beliefs led her to revisit the race from a less emotional perspective, recognize the realities of what went wrong (questionable nutrition in the days prior to the race and not enough rest), and plan for success in the future. (And a quick postscript: seven months later, she ran another marathon—twenty-five minutes faster than on that bad day!)

friends, or a medical diagnosis that changes everything about the way you see yourself and the world. I've seen cancer survivors come back to scale mountain peaks, and broken relationships blossom into new, healing ones through physical fitness.

One tool we have at our disposal is acceptance. It's probably the easiest word to say and the hardest thing to do.

So how do you cope? You will feel a sense of loss. If anybody was to take a direction, to walk down a path, or commit to a journey of effort and exploration they expected to end with a certain result and not reach it, it would be normal to feel a sense of loss.

If a small setback deserves some time to reframe the situation, then a big setback deserves a larger amount of time to reframe. So how do you move forward in a practical way? It's not easy to suggest that somebody who found the activity of their dreams accept that they can't put any weight on their feet for the next three months, and that they take up swimming. If we can take a direction that we didn't choose but that was chosen for us and ask, "What can I do about this situation?" we may find strength inside ourselves that we never knew existed. Sometimes the depth of the loss must be matched with something approaching defiance to enable us to take charge and move ahead.

One example I'll never forget was watching a soldier fall from a climbing rope in a gym. He fell twenty feet to the ground and sustained a double femur fracture. Even though his doctor had not come to any conclusions, there was significant doubt as to whether this soldier would be able to continue his career. But in a matter of days, he hauled himself back into the same gym, the same exercise class, and proceeded to roll his wheelchair to the very same rope where he fell. He did pull-ups on the rope. Some people would say that was a crazy move. In this case it was probably risky—had he fallen again, he could have hurt himself very badly. But what it meant to him in the moment was that he was able to accept both what had happened and that this setback, as great as it seemed, would not control his ability to do something for himself. Stories like this are a humbling reminder of the possibilities to not only endure the setbacks, but to succeed beyond them.

OPPORTUNITIES: TURNING CHALLENGES AND SETBACKS AROUND

All athletes go through setbacks. For professional athletes, a setback can feel like a very personal failure because so much of who they are is tied to their athletic performance. The key to a lifetime of outdoor fitness is to keep perspective on the right goals—you might start out focusing on a race time goal, but then rework that goal to simply wanting within yourself to race to the best of your ability.

I've seen athletes sometimes make their biggest gains and experience their greatest successes right after an illness or a long layoff due to injury. Improvement, in fitness and in any other aspect of life, is not a linear phenomenon.

Some challenges feel overwhelming, like extended unemployment. Outdoor fitness costs nearly nothing, save for the cost of good gear. By working out regularly while you're job-searching, you can keep up your energy, positive focus, and confidence. If you're the caretaker of a sick parent or child, you can do push-ups in the living room while you're tending to them. Be creative and see that no matter what challenge you're facing, you can always fit in a way to be active and to preserve the fitness gains you've made.

If you can't walk, lift hand weights. If you're injured, figure out what you can do right now to improve your health, even if it's only eating the healthiest you can until you get back on your feet. No matter what, remember that this struggle will pass, and you will be a stronger athlete—and a stronger person—for having gone the distance.

epilogue: fit by nature

For many years, I've come to associate the act of going outdoors with happiness. I enjoy doing some morning exercises at a gym or inside my home, but nothing lifts my spirits like going outside. At times this has translated to getting as far away as I can from any semblance of civilization so that I could better experience nature, or so I thought at the time. But I took it to extremes at times. On an expedition to Mount McKinley shortly after my father passed away, I wanted to escape. I climbed solo from the high camp, only to realize that instead of being connected to anything, I felt cold and lonely. At one point I saw a small bird descending from the sky. When he stopped, he couldn't fly again. I took him in my hand to warm him up in my jacket and he started to look better, but then after fluttering his wings a bit, he suddenly stopped and died right there in front of me. I felt very, very disconnected from nature at that moment.

I remember getting back from that trip and landing in Seattle on a Sunday morning in June, taking a run around Green Lake, one of our beautiful parks, and realizing that I was surrounded by the very thing I'd tried to escape from: lush trees, grass, flowers everywhere, people running, cycling, walking dogs, and playing with children, rowers on the water, a soccer match being played, and a collective immeasurable sense of enjoyment. Mount McKinley, a thousand miles away, was a cold and desolate place with thin air, no plants, and few people. In contrast, getting from my home to Green Lake took less than five minutes—and the connectedness to nature was utterly complete.

That's one lesson I hope you can take from this book—that connectedness to nature is one of the things that makes us truly alive in the world, but that you don't have to journey far to find it. Outdoor exercise has led me to come full circle to an idea I embraced as a child: simply put, playing outside is *fun*!

I can travel a long distance for a great adventure, and I've done that many times, but I can also experience the intensity of the natural world right in the city where I live—or any place in the world that I visit.

I was in a fitness class that my friend Paul was leading and someone asked a question about why we were doing this outside. Without missing a beat, he replied, "It's organic. If you have your hand on the grass, you are connected to your planet. You are connected to the greatest source of energy you could ever know. It's good for you, and you'll get a better workout than if you are on the treadmill watching TV."

Are there days when I don't feel like it? Yes—at least when I'm getting started. But I've also rarely finished a workout without feeling more alive and energized than I did when I began. There will inevitably be a few standoffs with the alarm clock and that infamous snooze button, or the odd day when things get in the way of going outside, but that's okay. What I've learned is that I'm not restricted by place and time, energy level or motivation. Like a river or stream, I go with the flow...and I generally get where I'm going.

You're at the beginning of a wonderful journey. As you experience your own adventure with outdoor fitness, consider sharing your thoughts with us at www.adventx.com. We'd love to hear about where you've found your own outdoor playground, what you're training for, what goals you've set for yourself, and maybe even some new exercise or class concepts that you've derived from your training. Regardless of where you started when you first picked up this book, you're in the midst of experiencing the gift of training yourself to be a stronger and fitter athlete, and a more awake and aware human being. The outdoors will change your life. Best wishes for your journey.

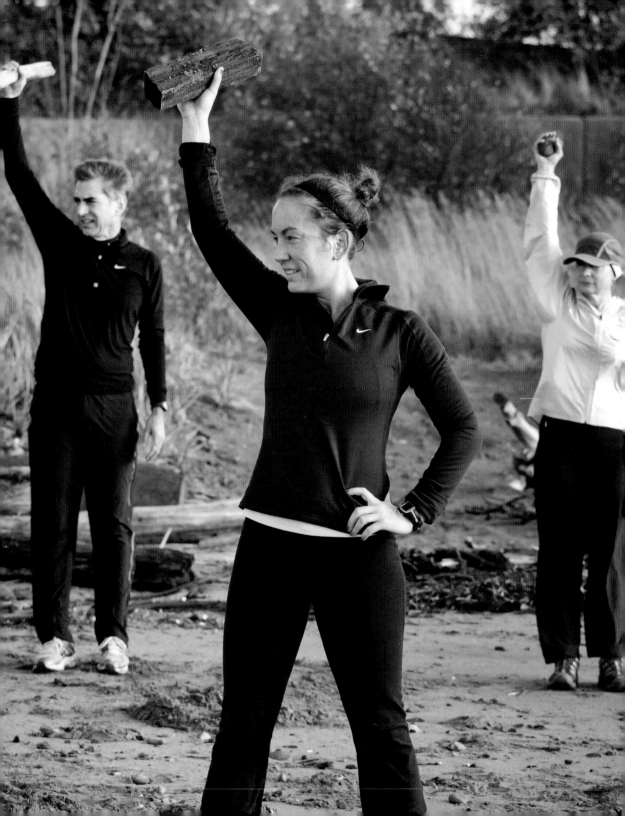

appendix a:
compendium
of exercises

What follows is the full compendium of exercises used throughout this book, with full descriptions and photographs of all of the major exercises you will use in this program. As you move through each week of workouts, you'll notice that many of the exercises below are variations on basic movements— so don't worry if this list seems overwhelming at first. Take the time to practice each movement with good form and good body alignment, and you'll find that you're able to learn how to perform these exercises correctly.

The exercises below are grouped according to the major goal of the exercise: core, lower body, upper body, whole body, and drills. The full index at the front of this section lists all of the exercises and their variations, along with the page numbers where you will see them explained in greater detail.

The following exercises can be found in the Home Stretch section (page 75):

The following exercises can be found in the Daily Dozen section (page 67):

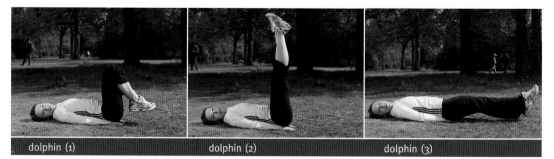

dolphin (1) dolphin (2) dolphin (3)

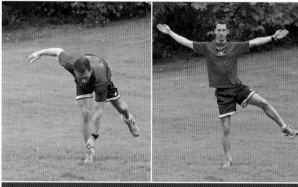

lawnmower pull (1) lawnmower pull (2)

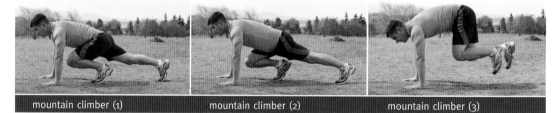

mountain climber (1) mountain climber (2) mountain climber (3)

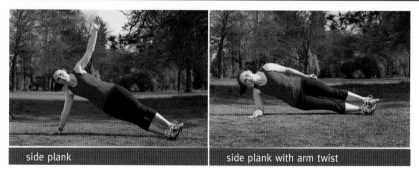

side plank side plank with arm twist

CORE

Dolphin

Start by lying down on your back. In a 3-count motion, bring your knees to your chest, then extend your legs up to a 90-degree angle with your body, then lower your legs to just above the ground, keeping your legs straight during the downward motion. Perform the recommended number of repetitions and then reverse the motion, pushing your bent knees out and straightening the legs, then lifting the legs to 90 degrees before bending the knees close to the chest.

Lawnmower Pull

Stand on your right leg, with your left leg trailing. Reach down with your left arm and imagine you're grabbing hold of a lawnmower starter. With all of your weight driving through your right heel for balance, imagine you have roots extending from your heel into the ground. Make sure your spine is in a neutral position. "Pull" the lawnmower cord up to an imaginary point, with your arm rising up level to your shoulder while you raise your body to an upright position, standing on your right leg. This exercise is a bigger challenge than it seems, so take it slow and find your balance and core strength as you move through the movement.

Mountain Climber

Start in a Plank position (see below). Move your right foot up so that it is directly below your right shoulder. This is your starting position. From there, switch your feet so that your right foot is extended behind you, and your left foot is beneath your left shoulder. The switch is done as one movement, so both legs will be off the ground at the same time. (Variation: Ranger Crawls.)

Plank and Plank Variations

The Plank is designated as a Daily Dozen exercise (page 73). Here we've included two Plank variations: the Side Plank and the Side Plank with Arm Twist:

Side Plank. From a Plank position, raise your right arm off the ground and tilt your body upward, reaching up with your right arm toward the sky. Your body weight will be supported by your feet and either your left hand (arm straight) or left elbow, whichever is more comfortable. Beginners will want to have both feet on the ground, toe to heel; more advanced athletes will be able to "stack" their

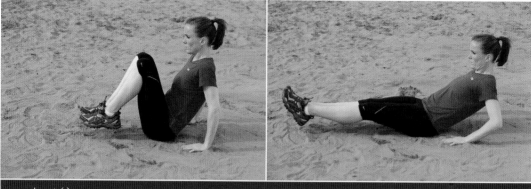

push-out (1) push-out (2)

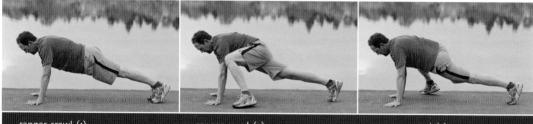

ranger crawl (1) ranger crawl (2) ranger crawl (2)

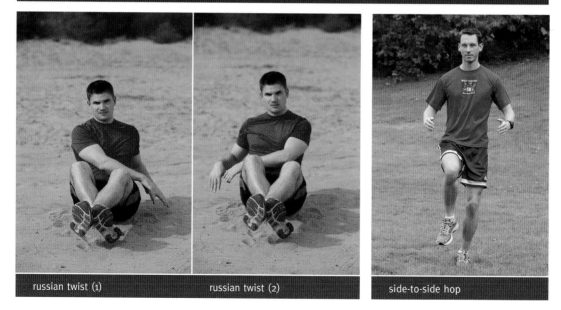

russian twist (1) russian twist (2) side-to-side hop

feet so that the left foot is on the ground with the right foot directly on top of the left foot. Hold for the designated period of time, then switch sides.

Side Plank with Arm Twist. From the side Plank position with right arm extended to the sky, reach your right arm down underneath your torso as far as it will go, while maintaining a strong core. Rotate your arm back up so that it is reaching to the sky. Do all of your repetitions on this side, then switch sides.

Push-out
Start by sitting on the ground with knees bent. Support your weight by placing your hands behind you on the ground. Push your legs out in front of you, a few inches above the ground, and push back into the starting position. Advanced variation: instead of having your hands on the ground for support, perform a "rowing" motion with your arms, pulling your arms back as your legs push forward.

Ranger Crawl
This is a variation on Mountain Climber. Starting in Plank position, move your right leg to just below your right shoulder, then back to Plank position. Alternate this movement by putting your left leg below your left shoulder, always making sure to have your trailing leg on the ground.

Russian Twist
Start in the same starting position as with Push-outs, described above. For beginners, keep your feet on the ground and lean back so that your upper body is at about a 45-degree angle to the ground. Keep your core strong as you reach both hands to the left, twisting your torso as far as is comfortable, and reverse direction. (Advanced variation: lift your feet a few inches off the ground.)

Side-to-Side Hop
In sand or dirt, draw a large plus sign (+) with your foot. Jump side to side, up and back, first on two legs, then one leg at a time. The jumping pattern is as follows: diagonal from lower left corner to upper right corner, across to upper left, diagonally down to the right hand corner, and across to the lower left hand corner. Remember to do this exercise in both directions.

Skydiver

Lie down on your stomach with your arms extended out and to the side, like a skydiver. Inhale and gently raise your arms, legs and head off the ground. Hold this position for the designated amount of time, then gently bring your arms, legs, and head back down to the ground.

Squat and Reach

Stand with your feet about shoulder-width apart. Perform a basic Squat, going down far enough to touch your hands to the ground if you can. From there, push up through your heels, extend your legs, and reach your hands up to the sky. Look for the stretch in your abdominal muscles; that will indicate that you're really getting the full benefits of the stretch.

Squat Thruster

Start in a Push-up position. Keeping your upper body and core strong, jump with your feet into a Squat position, keeping your hands on the ground. Your knees can go either directly underneath your torso or out to each side—whichever is more comfortable. **Variation**: The Wolfgang. Try doing this exercise by alternating the ending position of your knees—one time out to the side, the next time directly underneath your torso. Your knees will make the shape of the letter W—a tribute to adventX's resident physical therapist, Wolfgang Brolley, who reviewed all of the exercises in this book.

Superman

The starting position is on all fours, with your weight supported on hands and knees. Extend your left arm straight out in front of you, while simultaneously pushing your right leg back so that the leg is straight and in line with your torso. Hold for 15 (beginner), 30 (intermediate), or 60 (advanced) seconds. The advanced variation for this exercise is to start in a Plank position, and from there lift your left arm and right leg off the ground. Switch sides.

Thirsty Bird

Stand on one leg, hands up in the air, palms touching. Lean forward gently and slowly until you've made a capital T with your body. Your start position is straight up and down, while in the finish position your trailing leg, arms, and body will all be at 90-degree angles. Note that it's very important to do this movement slowly because the load on the hamstring muscles as you rise

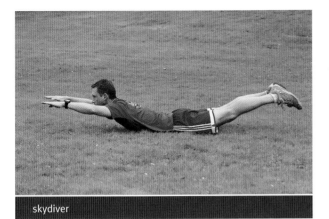

skydiver

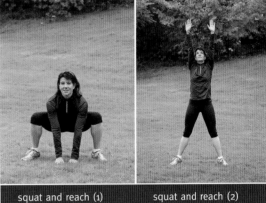

squat and reach (1)   squat and reach (2)

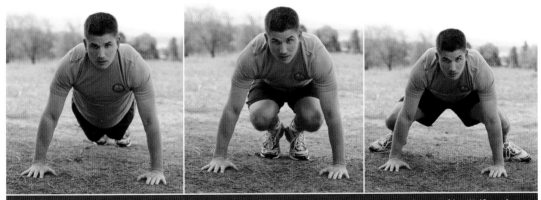

squat thruster (1)   squat thruster (2)   squat thruster (the Wolfgang)

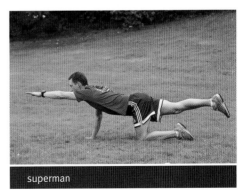

superman

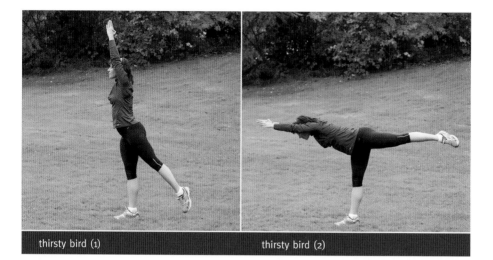

thirsty bird (1) | thirsty bird (2)

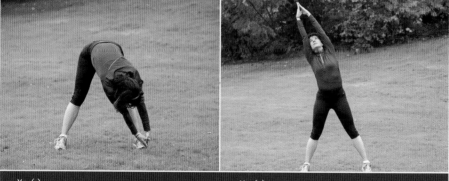

Xs (1) | Xs (2)

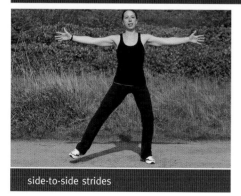

side-to-side strides

up from the 90-degree position is so great that if you accelerate, you risk straining the hamstrings. This is a fantastic hamstring exercise as well as a great balance-builder.

Xs

Stand up straight with your feet about 12 to 18 inches apart. Reach down with both hands to touch your left toe (you can bend your knees if needed), and from there stretch as high as you can above your right shoulder—as though you are trying to touch the right upper corner of the sky. Do all of your repetitions on this side, and then reverse the movement, going from the right toe to the left upper corner of the sky, to form a complete X with your body motion.

DRILLS

The Cal Ripken Special (Baseball Diamond Drill)

Described in detail in the El Rapido Cornerstone Workout (Week 7), page 157.

Illinois Agility Drill

Described in detail in the El Rapido Cornerstone Workout (Week 7), page 154.

Shuttle Run

Described in detail in the Put It to the Test Cornerstone Workout (Week 4), page 116.

Side-to-Side Strides (Running Warmup)

Stride sideways in a skipping motion, leading with your right leg. Stride for 15 to 20 seconds, and then turn 180 degrees to the other side and stride with your left leg leading for another 15 to 20 seconds.

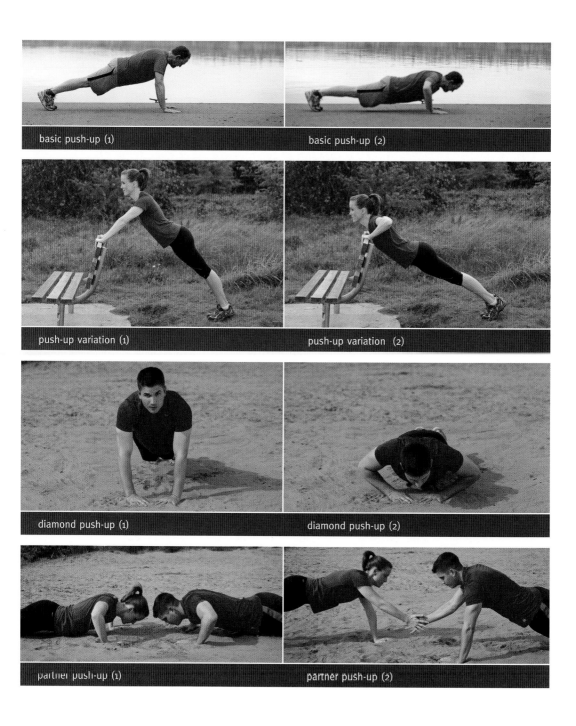

basic push-up (1)

basic push-up (2)

push-up variation (1)

push-up variation (2)

diamond push-up (1)

diamond push-up (2)

partner push-up (1)

partner push-up (2)

UPPER BODY

Key Exercise: Push-up

Push-ups feel hard sometimes because you have to overcome a tremendous amount of resistance to push your entire body weight off the ground. The trick is to reduce the resistance by either changing the angle of your body by doing the Push-ups from your knees, or leaning against something: a picnic bench, a rock, a log, a railing, a wall. You can also use a slope, such as the slope of a hill. What's key is to complete the Push-up. To change the angle to make them harder, you can perform **decline push-ups** by elevating your feet on a log or bench. The most advanced Push-up is a handstand Push-up with legs in the air, which few people can perform.

Basic Push-up Technique: Start with palms and toes on the ground, with arms straight, a straight back, neutral spine, and a strong core (a modified Plank position). Your fingers should be pointing forward and should be shoulder-width apart. Maintaining that position, inhale as you slowly lower your body to within a couple of inches off the ground, and exhale as you push up. Be sure not to bend your neck down as you perform this movement; think of the top of your head, your shoulder blades, and your tailbone staying in one perfect line. If you'd like to test your posture, place a wooden dowel on top of your body as you perform the movement to be sure you're keeping your spine straight.

Other Push-up variations

Diamond Push-up
Perform a regular Push-up but with your hands in a "diamond" shape, placing your thumbs and index fingers together directly underneath your chest.

Partner Push-up
This is a great variation when you're working out with others. Start in the regular Push-up position, with a partner in the same position facing you. Each of you will perform a Push-up, and at the top of the movement, clap your right hands together. On the next repetition, clap your left hands together.

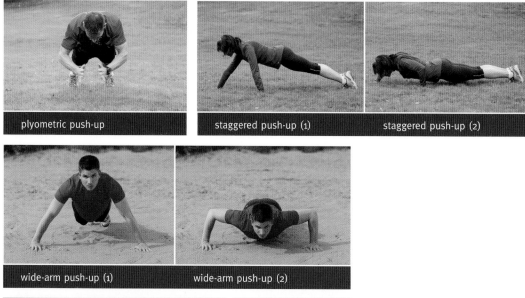

plyometric push-up   staggered push-up (1)   staggered push-up (2)

wide-arm push-up (1)   wide-arm push-up (2)

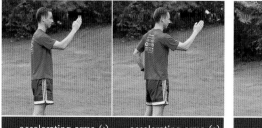 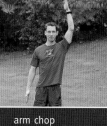

accelerating arms (1)   accelerating arms (2)   arm chop

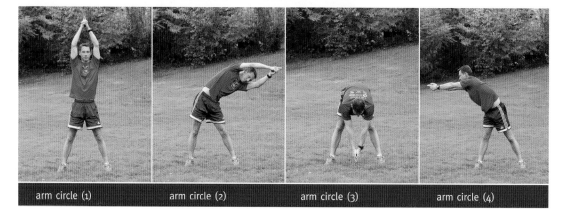

arm circle (1)   arm circle (2)   arm circle (3)   arm circle (4)

Plyometric Push-up (Clappers)
Among the hardest Push-up variations, this exercise is performed by lowering yourself into the normal Push-up position, then pushing your body up with enough force to take your hands off the ground and clap them together before ending in the normal Push-up ending position. You can also do plyometric Push-ups on an incline, using a log or a park bench, to decrease the resistance.

Staggered Push-up
Perform a regular Push-up, but with your hands in a "staggered" position, that is, with your left hand placed on the ground above your head and your right hand on the ground just outside your right shoulder. Switch arms midway through the set.

Wide-Arm Push-up
Perform a regular Push-up, but with your hands placed wide on the ground, a few inches wider than your shoulders.

Accelerating Arms
The goal of this exercise is to get the body warmed up for a full range of motion. In a standing position, bend your elbows and move your arms back and forth first slowly, then more quickly, then as quickly as you can.

Arm Chop
The purpose of this exercise is to warm up the shoulder joint. With arms straight, move them up and down from your shoulders in a chopping motion at a moderate pace. Take care not to move your arms too fast—move deliberately and purposefully.

Arm Circle
This exercise promotes good balance and will stretch parts of the body that almost never get stretched. Place your hands together, with arms extended above your head. Clasp your hands together and then point your index fingers up. Draw the biggest circle you can with your arms by first squatting down and then extending up, reaching your arms out as wide and high as you can to draw a huge circle.

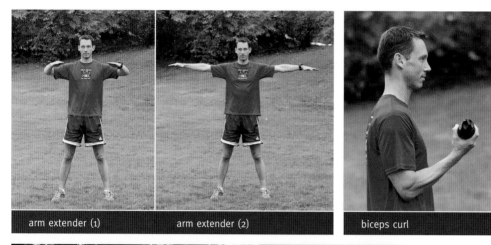

arm extender (1)   arm extender (2)   biceps curl

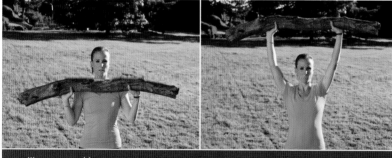

military press (1)   military press (2)

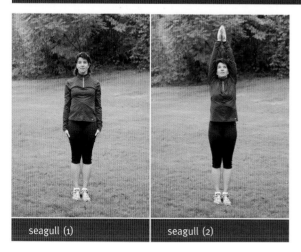

seagull (1)   seagull (2)

Arm Extender

This is a 4-count exercise to warm up the arms and upper/middle back. Bend your elbows and move them as far behind your back as you can, looking for a squeezing sensation in your shoulder blades. Do this three times. On the fourth count, perform the same movement but with arms fully extended.

Biceps Curl

Holding a rock, a weight, or an exercise band, slowly bend the elbow only, contracting the biceps muscles as you lift the weight. The only part of your body that should move during this exercise is the elbow—be sure to have a strong core and to never swing your back (that's an indication that you're attempting to lift too much weight).

Military Press

Holding rocks, weights, or the handles of a resistance band or even a small log, extend your arms directly above your head, meeting in the middle when your arms are fully extended. Slowly lower your arms to the starting position.

Pull-up

Hanging from a bar, slowly pull yourself up so that your chin reaches the bar. You can have your hands in a variety of positions for this exercise: over-handed, under-handed, wide grip, or narrow grip. Try **assisted pull-ups** if this is too difficult for you: perform pull-ups with a partner holding your feet and press your feet into their hands for assistance. Another variation to try if you're working your way up to regular pull-ups is **negative pull-ups**: have your partner help you lift into the upper position of a pull-up, with chin at the same level as the bar, and slowly lower your body under your own control until you are in the pull-up starting position.

Seagull

This is a shoulder flexibility exercise. Standing upright with your arms straight at your sides, raise both arms at once, in a semicircle, touching the backs of your hands when they meet at the top. Take care to do this exercise slowly and deliberately—there's no value in trying to do it too quickly, and in fact you could injure your shoulders if you move too fast.

Sun God

This is a variation on Arm Circles. Perform Arm Circles in both directions, first to the side, then to the front, then with arms stretched up above your head, moving from small to large circles and then back to small circles again.

Triceps Dip

With hands on the edge of a park bench, picnic bench, step, or log, move your legs forward just enough so that your bottom is very close to the step, but not touching it. Bend your elbows to lower your body down, and straighten them while exhaling to push yourself back up to the start position. **Variation:** if no bench or step is available, you can perform Triceps Dips on the ground simply by sitting on the ground with hands on the ground about six inches behind you, knees bent, and feet on the ground in front of you.

Upright Row

This is a great exercise for forearms, shoulders, and back. Stand upright, feet shoulder width apart, holding a light weight in both hands or a rock in each. With your palms facing your body, lift the weights in a vertical plane until your hands are at the level of your shoulders. Your elbows will naturally point out to the sides. Slowly lower the weights.

LOWER BODY

Key Exercise: Squat

The Squat is the king of lower-body exercises: they're underestimated and rarely performed in a fully correct manner. Your task is to do the best Squats you've ever done. The explanation will help you to learn how.

Start by standing straight, with a neutral spine, good posture, and weight balanced equally on your legs. Take a deep breath, tighten your torso and abdominals, and imagine that somebody is going to climb on your shoulders. Your muscles should have a relaxed tension, with weight distributed evenly between heels and balls of your feet, and a slight bend in your knees as well.

You should also feel some tension in your abdominal muscles; focus on the tension coming from about an inch or two behind your belly button.

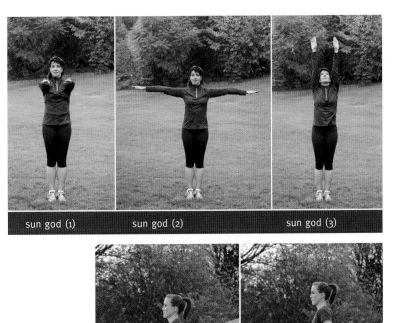

sun god (1)   sun god (2)   sun god (3)

triceps dip (1)   triceps dip (2)

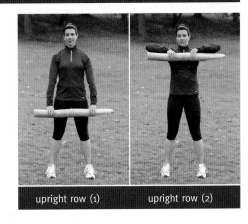

upright row (1)   upright row (2)

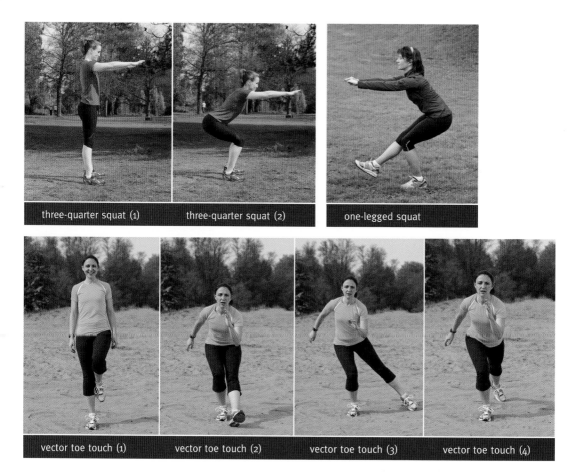

three-quarter squat (1)   three-quarter squat (2)   one-legged squat

vector toe touch (1)   vector toe touch (2)   vector toe touch (3)   vector toe touch (4)

Imagine you have a tail and that it's tucked between your legs, so that you're tilting your body slightly forward. You should feel balanced, strong, and confident.

When you've achieved the right starting position, take a few deep breaths. Repeat until you feel completely centered. Place your body weight on your heels and drive your hips backward as you bend your knees, keeping your back straight. By driving the hips backward, you'll perform a more balanced Squat than you would by simply bending your knees (which tends to create a forward lean in your upper body). Press your weight into your heels as you rise up from the Squat position.

Squat variations

Three-Quarter Squat
Described in detail in the Daily Dozen (page 69).

One-Legged Squat
Place one leg in front of the other, just slightly off the ground. If necessary, position a log, bench, or step behind you for support. With all of your body weight on one leg, slowly push your bottom back and bend your knee to whatever point is comfortable for you (the goal is to be able to lower your bottom to just above the log or bench behind you). Slowly raise your body as you exhale.

Sumo Squat
Described in detail in the Daily Dozen (page 71).

Vector Toe Touch
This is a variation on a One-Legged Squat. Perform a set of three One-Legged Squats on your left leg, with your right leg first extended in front of you (12 o'clock), then to the side (3 o'clock) and then behind you (6 o'clock). Repeat on the other side, with your left leg in the 12, 9, and 6 o'clock positions. Beginners can lightly touch the right toe to the ground when performing the One-Legged Squat; the more advanced variation is to keep the right leg off the ground during the entire movement.

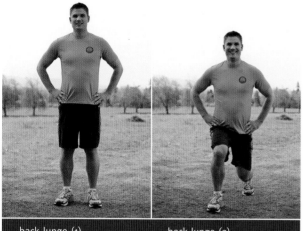

back lunge (1)   back lunge (2)

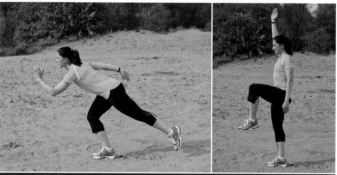

backwards lunge to high knee (1)   backwards lunge to high knee (2)

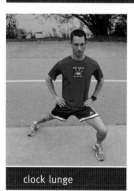

clock lunge

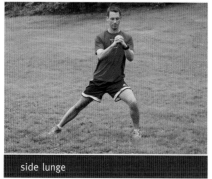

side lunge

Key Exercise: Lunge

The other key lower-body exercise in the adventX program is the Lunge. The basic Lunge is described in detail in the Daily Dozen (page 70). Below you'll find four variations on the basic lunge movement.

Lunge variations

Back Lunge
Perform a Lunge by keeping your left leg stationary and stepping directly behind you with your right leg into a lunge position. Step back to the starting position and reverse legs.

Backwards Lunge to High Knee
Start in lunge position, with your right leg back. Pushing off the right leg, rise up, performing a high knee movement with the right leg. Think of mimicking a huge runner's step. The movement should be slow and smooth, with emphasis on raising the knee high and maintaining good balance all the way through. It's useful here to have a pause at each phase of the movement: a pause at the top, and a second pause at the bottom.

Clock Lunge
This Lunge variation is particularly good for the iliotibial band. Keeping your left leg stationary, step into a Lunge with your right leg tracing the shape of a clock: first step directly in front of your body (12 o'clock), then to your right side at the 1, 2, 3, 4, 5, and 6 o'clock positions. Switch legs so your right leg becomes the stationary leg as you step your left leg directly back to the 6 o'clock position, then to your left in the 7, 8, 9, 10, 11, and 12 o'clock positions. Repeat in the counterclockwise direction (left leg first, from 12 to 7, following each number; then right leg back to 6 o'clock, 5, 4 to 1 and then 12 again).

Side Lunge
Begin by standing straight with legs and feet together. Perform a Lunge by stepping directly out to the side with your right leg, taking care to keep your upper body directly above your pelvis—don't bend forward. Lower your knee into a Lunge and then press back up to the starting position. Switch legs.

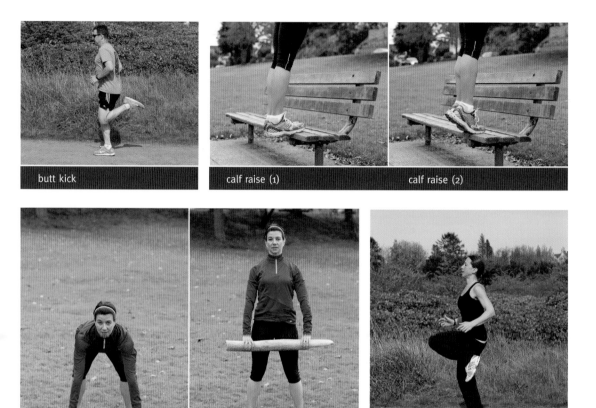

butt kick

calf raise (1)

calf raise (2)

deadlifts (1)

deadlifts (2)

high knees

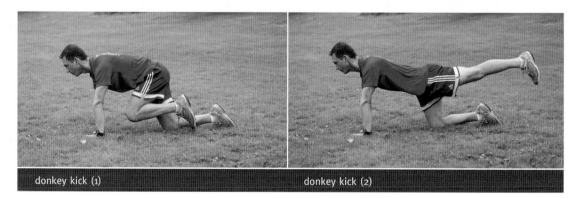

donkey kick (1)

donkey kick (2)

Ankle Alphabet

Standing with one arm supporting you against a tree or wall, trace the alphabet with the toe of one foot, then the other foot, for an excellent ankle warmup.

Butt Kick

Jog forward, pushing your heels back as close to your bottom as possible as you take your steps. Try to literally kick your butt. This is a great warmup for running.

Calf Raise

Step onto a stair, log, or bench, with your toes on the stair and your heels extended out beyond the stair. Stand on your tiptoes and then lower back to the starting position (foot in neutral position). Take care not to lower your heels below your toes—that can put too much stress on the calf muscles.

Deadlifts

Place a light or medium weight or two rocks on the ground in front of you, just beyond your toes. Bend down with core muscles engaged to grasp the weights. Keeping your legs straight if possible, imagine using your hamstrings to lift your upper body while holding the weights. Lift up to a standing position.

High Knees

Jog forward, lifting your knees as high as they will go with each step. You can hold your hands out, palms down, at waist level, and try to touch your knees to your palms with every step. This is an excellent warmup for running; we normally will do it in tandem with Butt Kicks.

Donkey Kick

Start on all fours. Bring your right knee in toward your chest, and then kick it straight out behind you, raising your leg a few inches above your torso. Do the recommended number of repetitions, and then switch sides.

Leg Swing

To warm up your legs before an intense effort, swing one leg in three planes: forward and backward, side to side, and on an angle as though you

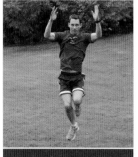

power hop

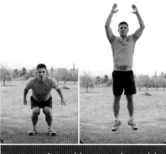

power jump (1)   power jump (2)

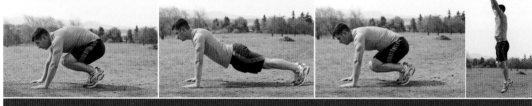

burpee (1)   burpee (2)   burpee (3)   burpee (4)

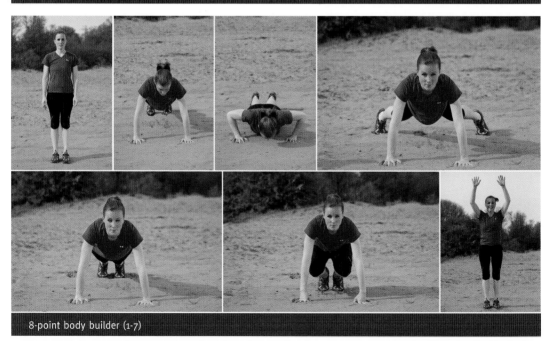
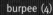

8-point body builder (1-7)

are trying to kick a soccer ball. Do 10 leg swings in each of the three planes, then switch legs.

Power Hop
Hop up and down, trying to gain as much upward motion as you can with each hop. **Variation:** Side-to-Side Hops—instead of staying in one place, hop first to your left and then to your right.

Power Jump
Jump upwards and land on your feet with soft knees. Variations include **Star Jumps** (jump upwards, spreading your legs in midair and then landing in the normal power jump landing position) and **Scissor Jumps** (starting the jump in a lunge position and switching the position of your feet in midair, so that if you start in a lunge position with left leg forward, you will land in a lunge position with right leg forward).

Skipping
Variations include skipping with high knees (pushing your knees up as far as they will go as you skip) and Gazelles (adding an arm movement to the high-knee movement, raising the left arm and right knee as high as they will go, and then switching sides).

WHOLE BODY

Key Exercise: Burpee
The most popular whole-body exercise in the adventX repertoire. This is a 4-count exercise. Start in a standing position. 1. Lower your hands to the ground, bending your knees. 2. Push your legs straight behind you into the starting position for a Push-up. 3. Perform a Squat Thruster, bringing your legs as close to your body as you can. 4. Perform a Power Jump, launching yourself off the ground, jumping up and extending your arms to the sky.

Burpee variations

8-Point Body Builder
An 8-count Burpee with an added Push-up and a scissor movement for the legs. Counts 1 and 2 are the same as the traditional Burpee, then in count 3, lower yourself into a Push-up; in count 4, complete the full Push-up. In count 5, jump with your legs out to each side so that your legs are in a scissor position; your arms will stay straight. In count 6, bring your legs back to the Push-up start position. Counts 7 and 8 correspond with counts 3 and 4 of a traditional Burpee: do a Squat Thruster followed by a Power Jump.

Projectile Burpee
Perform a traditional Burpee with one change—instead of doing a Power Jump, jump forward as far as you can.

Super Burpee
Perform a traditional Burpee with one change—instead of a regular Power Jump, do a bigger jump, trying to touch your knees to your hands.

Jump Rope
With or without a jump rope, perform a jump-rope movement for the allotted time—a great workout in its own right, or a great warmup for harder work to come.

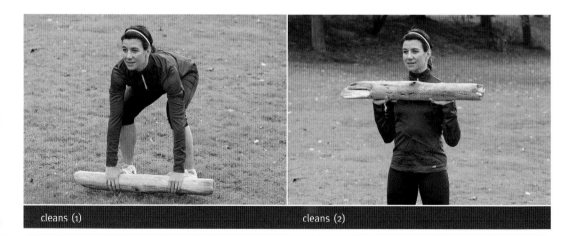

cleans (1)   cleans (2)

Cleans

Start in the same position as for the Deadlift, with a light or medium weight or two rocks on the ground in front of you. Bend down with a straight back and straight or slightly bent legs to pick up the weight or rocks from the ground. As you stand up, when the weights reach the level of your thighs, curl your biceps with palms facing outward so that by the time you are standing upright, the weights are at the level of your shoulders, with biceps fully engaged. Reverse the movement to place the weights back on the ground.

Jumping Jacks

A classic exercise that you probably remember from your childhood. Start in an upright standing position with legs together. In one count, jump and land with your legs out to each side, while bringing your arms above your head in a semicircle movement. On the second count, return to the starting position.

RUNNING WARMUPS

Backwards Walking and Running

Running or walking backwards is another great warmup exercise, particularly for the backs of your legs. Take care to look behind you and make sure that you can see where you are stepping.

High Knees

Jog forward, lifting your knees as high as they will go with each step. You can hold your hands out, palms down, at waist level and try to touch your knees to your palms with every step. This is an excellent warmup for running; we normally will do it in tandem with Butt Kicks.

Leg Swings

To warm up your legs before an intense effort, swing one leg in three planes: forwards and backwards, side to side, and on an angle as though you're trying to kick a soccer ball. Do 10 leg swings in each of the three planes, then switch legs.

appendix b:
sport-specific circuit training

In Week 3 (Super Circuits), we devoted the entire Cornerstone Workout to the concept of Circuit Training. If you're training for a specific sport, you may wish to alter your Circuit Training to incorporate movements that will strengthen the necessary skills for your sports. Below, you'll find examples of circuits to perform for specific sports.

Triathlon Circuit: The focus of this circuit is the shoulders, core, and legs.

Flutter Kicks (Lie on stomach with arms extended in front of your head. Flutter your legs up and down, as if swimming.)	
Steam Engines on Back	page 73
Push-ups	page 71
Squats	page 242
Ranger Crawls	page 231
Lunges	page 70
Side Plank	page 229
Burpees or 8-Point Body Builders	page 251

Cycling Circuit: This circuit emphasizes core strength, upper-body strength, and lateral side movement. Cyclists suffer from single-plane movement (moving in only one of the three major movement axes of the body) more than athletes in any other sport. Therefore, it's particularly important for cyclists to exercise parts of the body that don't normally get exercise on the bike.

Jumping Jacks	page 253
Steam Engines	page 68
Push-ups	page 71
Scissors	page 72
Ranger Crawls	page 231
Triceps Dips	page 242
Side Plank	page 229
Russian Twist	page 231

Running Circuit: This circuit is designed to increase flexibility, balance, and increase stabilizer muscles.

Jumping Jacks	page 253
Steam Engines	page 68
Push-ups	page 71
Calf Raises	page 249
Plank—hold for 1 minute	page 73
Squats	page 242
Side Lunges	page 247
Mountain Climbers	page 229

Mountaineering Circuit: This circuit is designed to increase core strength, exercise the body's full range of motion and movement, and increase balance.

Mountain Climbers	page 229
Plank	page 73
Push-ups	page 71
X Agility Drill	page 153
Toe Touchers	page 68
Vector Toe Touches	page 245
One-legged Squats	page 245
Clock Lunges	page 247

Skiing Circuit: This circuit focuses on core stability, lateral stability, agility, and explosiveness.

Side Lunges	page 247
Mountain Climbers	page 229
Squats	page 242
Steam Engines on Back	page 73
Plank	page 73
Push-outs	page 231
Burpees or a Burpee variation (Super Burpees or 8-Point Body Builders)	page 251
Russian Twists	page 231
Side-to-Side Hops (double or single leg)	page 231
Tuck Jumps (A variation on the Power Jump: perform a Power Jump and bring your knees up as far as you can.)	page 251

Backpacking Circuit: This circuit focuses on core strength, back strength, hip and lower leg strength, endurance, and stability.

Push-ups	page 71
Steam Engines on Back	page 73
Squats	page 242
Clock Lunges	page 247
Russian Twists	page 231
Vector Toe Touches	page 245
Sumo Squats	page 71
Crocodiles	page 72
Plank	page 73
Dolphin	page 229

appendix c:
adventX on-target questionnaire

This is the goal-setting questionnaire that all adventX athletes take when they begin their training, and again at regular intervals to gauge their progress and set new goals. Use this questionnaire as a tool for regular goal setting as well as checking in with yourself to see how your training is progressing from week to week, and from season to season.

Instructions and hints on completing this evaluation: The purpose of this evaluation is to become more aware of strengths and limitations and to explore possibilities. It is our belief that no one knows us as well as we know ourselves. We do not need an expert to tell us if we eat well, have good flexibility, climb flights of stairs all day, or complete a set of quality push-ups. Therefore, we begin the coaching process by asking you to evaluate your strengths and to consider your goals.

Evaluate your physiological strengths using the following scale.

1 — Significantly lacking
2 — Not satisfied
3 — Average
4 — Strong
5 — Very strong
6 — Couldn't be better

Cardiovascular Aerobic: Long endurance at moderate intensity.

1   2   3   4   5   6

Cardiovascular Anaerobic: Shorter efforts at high intensity.

1   2   3   4   5   6

Maximal Strength: Ability to create force.

1   2   3   4   5   6

Muscle Endurance: Ability to make repeated demands on specific muscle groups.

1   2   3   4   5   6

Agility: Explosive strength.

1   2   3   4   5   6

Balance (static).

1   2   3   4   5   6

Coordination.

1   2   3   4   5   6

Flexibility.

1   2   3   4   5   6

Power to weight ratio: Correct body composition.

1   2   3   4   5   6

Evaluate your lifestyle strengths using the following scale.

1 — Never
2 — Not so much
3 — Sometimes
4 — Mostly
5 — Nearly always
6 — Always

I eat nutritious and healthy food.

1   2   3   4   5   6

I eat sufficiently for my activities.

1   2   3   4   5   6

I eat breakfast every day.

1   2   3   4   5   6

I space my meals throughout the day.

1   2   3   4   5   6

I sleep well.

1   2   3   4   5   6

I drink sufficient water and am hydrated.

1   2   3   4   5   6

I take time to rest and relax.

1   2   3   4   5   6

I manage my stress well.

1   2   3   4   5   6

I am happy with my lifestyle.

1   2   3   4   5   6

My overall health is good.

1   2   3   4   5   6

Evaluate your enjoyment of fitness using the following scale.

1 — Absolutely not
2 — Not as much as I want
3 — Average
4 — Mostly
5 — Nearly always
6 — Absolutely

I enjoy training.

1   2   3   4   5   6

I feel that I am getting the results I want.

1   2   3   4   5   6

I have training objectives that motivate me.

1   2   3   4   5   6

I have goals that inspire me.

1   2   3   4   5   6

I have a plan to meet those goals.

1   2   3   4   5   6

I achieve my goals.

1   2   3   4   5   6

I am satisfied with my fitness.

1   2   3   4   5   6

I am the athlete I want to be.

1   2   3   4   5   6

Use the space below to elaborate on any aspects of fitness or lifestyle where you would like to experience different results. Remember that the past does not equal the future.

What are some of the results that you want to see as a result of your training?

What would you try if you knew you couldn't fail?

Indicate any goals that you have or wish to explore.

1 month:

3 months:

1 year:

5 years:

20 years or lifetime:

appendix d:
resources

The books and online resources listed below offer additional information about some of the subjects discussed in this book.

Running/Walking Training

Jeff Galloway, founder of the Galloway Marathon Training Program and author of numerous books on running and training, offers coaching and instruction on integrating walk breaks into running training: www.jeffgalloway.com.

Sports Nutrition

Clark, Nancy. *Nancy Clark's Food Guide for Marathoners*. Meyer & Meyer Sport LTD, 2007.
——. *Nancy Clark's Sports Nutrition Guidebook*, 4th ed. Human Kinetics, 2008.
Clark, Nancy, and Jenny Hegmann. *The Cyclist's Food Guide*. Sports Nutrition Publishers, 2005.
Coleman, Ellen. *Eating for Endurance*, 4th ed. Bull Publishing Company, 2003.
Coleman, Ellen, and Suzanne Nelson Steen. *Ultimate Sports Nutrition*, 2nd ed. Bull Publishing Company, 2000.
Dorfman, Lisa. *The Vegetarian's Sports Nutrition Guide*. John Wiley & Sons, 1999.
Dunford, Marie. *Fundamentals of Sport and Exercise Nutrition*. Human Kinetics, 2010.
——. *Nutrition for Sport and Exercise*. Thomson/Wadsworth, 2008.
——. *Sports Nutrition: A Practice Manual for Professionals*, 4th ed. SCAN Dietetic Practice Group, American Dietetic Association, 2006.

Eberle, Suzanne Girard. *Endurance Sports Nutrition*, 2nd ed. Human Kinetics, 2007.

Seebohar, Bob. *Nutrition Periodization for Endurance Athletes*. Bull Publishing Company, 2004.

Additional information on sports nutrition, as well as information on finding a board-certified sports dietician, can be found at www.scandpg.org (Sports, Cardiovascular, and Wellness Nutrition), the website for the sports nutrition practice group of the American Dietetic Association.

index

about the authors

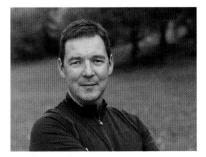

John Colver is an award-winning athletic coach, mountain guide, and former competitive cyclist. His outdoor training company, adventX, was named "Best Outdoor Fitness Program" by *Seattle* magazine, and Colver was nominated for KING-5 TV's "Best of Western Washington: Top Five Personal Trainers" award.

Colver founded adventX in 2003 and since that time has personally trained more than six hundred clients using the principles outlined in *Fit by Nature*. He has trained people ranging from age seventeen to seventy, from aspiring mountaineers and marathoners to casual athletes to those readying themselves for military training. Among his students are athletes who run anywhere from 5-kilometer to 100-mile races, compete in cycling and triathlon events, and summit major peaks, including Mount Everest.

It was as a teenager that Colver discovered his passion for outdoor recreation, endurance fitness training, and mountaineering. He has competed in more than three hundred road and track races in Europe, amassing fifty-two wins, including the Scottish 10-Mile Championship. He was a member of the Scottish National Cycling Team and raced for two leading French national teams. Colver has coached cycling in the United Kingdom and United States, raced in the expert category in mountain biking in the United States, and has completed fourteen marathons and two Ironman triathlons.

Colver served as a U.K. Parachute Regiment Officer and is a qualified military parachutist, emergency medical technician, and Wilderness First Responder. In addition to being an athletic coach, he is a professional mountain climbing instructor and guide with International Mountain Guides. He has guided seventy-five summit climbs of Mount Rainier and led summit expeditions to Aconcagua, the tallest peak in South America, as well as to Mount McKinley

(Denali), the tallest peak in North America. In 2008, he was the expedition leader for the U.S. Army's High Altitude Mountaineering Cognitive Study Research Group. He also leads expeditions on Mount Kilimanjaro.

Colver is a certified personal trainer with the American Council of Exercise and introduced outdoor fitness classes to athletic clubs throughout the greater Puget Sound region before creating his adventX brand. Currently, adventX leads training programs in Seattle and Colver presents clinics on outdoor fitness at companies such as Microsoft, Boeing, the American Lung Association, and REI. Colver lives in Seattle.

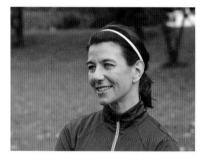 **M. Nicole Nazzaro** is a widely published sports and fitness writer who has written for *Sports Illustrated*'s English- and Chinese-language editions, *Runner's World*, the International Association of Athletics Federations, *American Track and Field* magazine, and the *San Francisco Chronicle*. She is an avid runner and a successful member of John Colver's adventX program in Seattle, where she has trained for a summit attempt of Mount Rainier and several marathons.

A graduate of Harvard College and the University of California–Berkeley's Graduate School of Journalism, Nazzaro taught sports journalism in China before working as *Sports Illustrated*'s China consultant for the 2008 Beijing Olympics. She worked with NBC Sports at the 2002, 2004, and 2006 Olympic Games and has served as a sports expert for the *International Herald Tribune*'s annual "Year in Sports" retrospective. She lives in Seattle.

Photographer **Sean Airhart** is a visual storyteller known for using a photojournalistic approach to help organizations communicate the humanistic side of their brand. He currently directs photography for one of the world's largest architectural firms, capturing the stories behind award-winning projects ranging from Fortune 500 headquarters to the world's top hospitals and universities. His work has been featured in numerous design publications such as *Architectural Record, Interior Design,* and *Contract* magazine. An avid cyclist and mountaineer, Sean lives in Seattle with his wife and son.

THE MOUNTAINEERS, founded in 1906, is a nonprofit outdoor activity and conservation club, whose mission is "to explore, study, preserve, and enjoy the natural beauty of the outdoors...." Based in Seattle, Washington, the club is now one of the largest such organizations in the United States, with seven branches throughout Washington State.

The Mountaineers sponsors both classes and year-round outdoor activities in the Pacific Northwest, which include hiking, mountain climbing, ski-touring, snowshoeing, bicycling, camping, canoeing and kayaking, nature study, sailing, and adventure travel. The club's conservation division supports environmental causes through educational activities, sponsoring legislation, and presenting informational programs.

All club activities are led by skilled, experienced volunteers, who are dedicated to promoting safe and responsible enjoyment and preservation of the outdoors.
If you would like to participate in these organized outdoor activities or the club's programs, consider a membership in The Mountaineers. For information and an application, write or call The Mountaineers, Club Headquarters, 7700 Sand Point Way NE, Seattle, WA 98115; 206-521-6001. You can also visit the club's website at www.mountaineers.org or contact The Mountaineers via email at clubmail@mountaineers.org.

The Mountaineers Books, an active, nonprofit publishing program of the club, produces guidebooks, instructional texts, historical works, natural history guides, and works on environmental conservation. All books produced by The Mountaineers Books fulfill the club's mission.

Visit **www.mountaineersbooks.org** to find details about all our titles and the latest author events, as well as videos, web clips, links, and more!

The Mountaineers Books
1001 SW Klickitat Way, Suite 201, Seattle, WA 98134
800-553-4453
mbooks@mountaineersbooks.org

The Mountaineers Books is proud to be a corporate sponsor of The Leave No Trace Center for Outdoor Ethics, whose mission is to promote and inspire responsible outdoor recreation through education, research, and partnerships. The Leave No Trace program is focused specifically on human-powered (nonmotorized) recreation.

Leave No Trace strives to educate visitors about the nature of their recreational impacts, as well as offer techniques to prevent and minimize such impacts. Leave No Trace is best understood as an educational and ethical program, not as a set of rules and regulations.

For more information, visit www.lnt.org, or call 800-332-4100.

OTHER TITLES YOU MIGHT ENJOY FROM
THE MOUNTAINEERS BOOKS

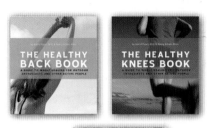

The Healthy Back Book
The Healthy Knees Book
Astrid Pujari, M.D, and Nancy Schatz Alton
Accessible advice for active individuals

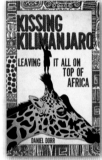

Kissing Kilimanjaro: Leaving It All on Top of Africa
Daniel Dorr
A humorous and inspirational account of climbing Africa's highest peak

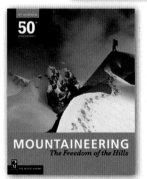

Mountaineering: The Freedom of the Hills, 8th edition
The Mountaineers
The essential mountaineering reference

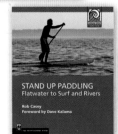

Stand Up Paddling: Flatwater to Surf and Rivers
Rob Casey
A comprehensive guide to this fun and fast growing sport

THE MOUNTAINEERS BOOKS
www.mountaineersbooks.org
800-553-4453